LIVING BETTER

WITH

DIABETES

AS A VEGAN

Transforming Health Through Nourishing Plant-Based Choices and Mindful Living for Optimal Diabetes Management

Catherine Clarkson

Contents

Introduction:

Embracing a Vegan Lifestyle with Diabetes

Living with diabetes can be a challenging journey, requiring constant attention to diet, lifestyle, and overall well-being. In recent years, a growing body of evidence suggests that embracing a vegan lifestyle can be a powerful and positive choice for individuals managing diabetes. This book explores the intersection of veganism and diabetes, delving into the reasons behind this lifestyle choice, its potential benefits, and practical considerations for those seeking to navigate the intricate landscape of diabetic health.

Embracing a Vegan Lifestyle with Diabetes

In the quest for better diabetes management, many individuals are turning to a vegan lifestyle as a holistic approach to address their health concerns. Embracing a vegan diet involves abstaining from consuming animal products, including meat, dairy, and eggs, and adopting a plant-based approach to nutrition. For those with diabetes, this decision is often motivated by the desire to improve blood sugar control, enhance overall health, and reduce the risk of complications associated with the condition.

One of the primary reasons individuals with diabetes consider embracing a vegan lifestyle is the potential impact on blood sugar levels. Plant-based diets, when well-balanced and thoughtfully planned, have been shown to contribute to improved glycemic control. The abundance of fiber, vitamins, and minerals in plant-based foods can positively influence insulin sensitivity and reduce the risk of sudden spikes in blood sugar. As we delve into the intricacies of this dietary choice, it becomes apparent that the synergy between a vegan lifestyle and diabetes management goes beyond glycemic control alone.

Vegans often emphasize a whole-food, plant-based approach, rich in fruits, vegetables, legumes, and whole grains. These nutrient-dense foods provide essential vitamins and minerals that contribute to overall health and well-being. The emphasis on plant-based sources of protein and healthy fats aligns with the principles of a balanced diet, which is crucial for individuals with diabetes aiming to achieve and maintain a healthy weight.

Beyond the physiological benefits, embracing a vegan lifestyle with diabetes is also a conscientious choice with environmental and ethical considerations. The production of plant-based foods generally has a lower environmental impact compared to animal agriculture, contributing to sustainability efforts and reducing one's carbon footprint. Ethically, adopting a vegan lifestyle aligns with the values of compassion and kindness towards animals, making it a choice that extends beyond personal health.

However, the decision to embrace a vegan lifestyle with diabetes is not one-size-fits-all. It requires careful consideration of individual health needs, preferences, and potential challenges. Proper planning is essential to ensure that a vegan diet meets all nutritional requirements, especially for individuals with diabetes who need to monitor their carbohydrate intake, protein sources, and micronutrient levels.

For those navigating diabetes and considering the shift to a vegan lifestyle, seeking guidance from healthcare professionals, including registered dietitians or nutritionists specializing in plant-based nutrition is crucial. These experts can provide personalized advice, helping individuals tailor their vegan diet to meet their specific health goals and manage their diabetes effectively.

As we embark on this exploration of embracing a vegan lifestyle with diabetes, it's essential to recognize that this choice is not about restriction or deprivation but rather about abundance and nourishment. The following sections will delve deeper into the nutritional foundations of a vegan diet, practical tips for meal planning, and strategies for navigating social situations and dining out. By understanding the intricacies of combining a vegan lifestyle with effective diabetes management, individuals can embark on a journey of improved health, mindful living, and a positive impact on the world around them.

Chapter 1:

Understanding Diabetes and Its Impact on Vegans

Diabetes is a complex and prevalent health condition that affects millions of individuals worldwide. Its management requires a nuanced understanding of various factors, including diet and lifestyle choices. This chapter aims to provide a comprehensive exploration of diabetes, considering its different types, prevalence, and the unique challenges and opportunities it presents for those who choose a vegan lifestyle.

Types of Diabetes: Overview and Prevalence

Diabetes mellitus is a group of metabolic disorders characterized by elevated blood sugar levels over an extended period. Understanding the different types of diabetes is fundamental to tailoring effective management strategies. The two main types are Type 1 and Type 2 diabetes, each with its distinct characteristics.

Type 1 Diabetes: Often diagnosed in childhood or adolescence, Type 1 diabetes results from the immune system mistakenly attacking and destroying insulin-producing beta cells in the pancreas. Individuals with Type 1 diabetes require insulin therapy for survival, as their bodies are unable to produce this crucial hormone. While Type 1 diabetes comprises a smaller percentage of diabetes cases, its impact on the lives of those affected is profound.

Type 2 Diabetes: This form of diabetes is more common and typically develops later in life, although it can also affect younger individuals. In Type 2 diabetes, the body either does not produce enough insulin or does not use it effectively, leading to insulin resistance. Lifestyle factors such as diet, physical activity, and genetics play a significant role in the development of Type 2 diabetes. Lifestyle modifications, oral medications, and, in some cases, insulin therapy are common approaches to managing Type 2 diabetes.

Prevalence and Global Impact: The global prevalence of diabetes has been steadily rising, fueled by factors such as sedentary lifestyles, unhealthy diets, and increasing obesity rates. According to the International Diabetes Federation (IDF), approximately 463 million adults were living with diabetes in 2019, a number expected to rise to 700 million by 2045 if current trends persist. These statistics underscore the urgency of understanding and addressing the impact of diabetes on various populations worldwide.

Vegans, like the general population, can be affected by both Type 1 and Type 2 diabetes. It's essential for individuals following a vegan lifestyle to be aware of their specific type of diabetes, as management approaches may vary. Additionally, the principles of a vegan diet can offer unique benefits for diabetes management, as explored in the next section.

Veganism and its Benefits for Diabetes Management

The decision to adopt a vegan lifestyle goes beyond personal preference; it can be a strategic choice for individuals managing diabetes. This section explores the intersection of veganism and diabetes, highlighting the potential benefits that a plant-based diet may offer for glycemic control, cardiovascular health, and overall well-being.

Impact on Glycemic Control: A well-planned vegan diet, rich in whole grains, fruits, vegetables, and legumes, can contribute to improved glycemic control for individuals with diabetes. The fiber content in plant-based foods slows down the absorption of glucose, preventing rapid spikes in blood sugar levels. Studies have shown that plant-based diets may enhance insulin sensitivity, potentially reducing the need for medication in some cases.

Cardiovascular Health: Diabetes is often associated with an increased risk of cardiovascular complications. Adopting a vegan lifestyle can positively impact cardiovascular health by reducing risk factors such as high blood pressure and elevated cholesterol levels. Plant-based diets are naturally low in saturated fats and cholesterol while being rich in antioxidants and anti-inflammatory compounds, supporting heart health.

Weight Management: Maintaining a healthy weight is crucial for individuals with diabetes, especially those with Type 2 diabetes. Vegan diets, when well-balanced, tend to be lower in calories and saturated fats, promoting weight loss or weight maintenance. The emphasis on whole, plant-based foods also provides essential nutrients without excessive caloric intake, supporting overall health.

Nutrient Density: Vegan diets, when carefully planned, can be highly nutrient-dense, providing essential vitamins, minerals, and antioxidants. This is particularly important for individuals with diabetes, as certain micronutrients play a role in glucose metabolism and overall well-being. Key nutrients such as fiber, magnesium, and vitamin C are abundant in plant-based foods and contribute to a holistic approach to diabetes management.

Ethical and Environmental Considerations: Beyond the individual health benefits, choosing a vegan lifestyle aligns with ethical and environmental values. Many individuals find motivation in reducing their impact on animal welfare and the environment. This holistic approach to well-being extends beyond personal health to encompass a broader perspective on interconnected global health.

While these potential benefits make a compelling case for adopting a vegan lifestyle with diabetes, it's essential to approach this dietary choice with careful consideration and individualization. Not all vegan diets are created equal, and factors such as meal planning, nutrient intake, and overall lifestyle play crucial roles in reaping the full spectrum of benefits.

Addressing Nutritional Concerns for Vegans with Diabetes

The intersection of veganism and diabetes requires careful attention to nutritional considerations. While a well-planned vegan diet can offer numerous health benefits, individuals with diabetes must be vigilant in meeting their specific nutritional needs. This section explores key nutritional concerns for vegans managing diabetes, offering insights into achieving a balanced and nourishing diet.

Protein Intake: Protein is an essential macronutrient, playing a crucial role in various bodily functions. For vegans with diabetes, ensuring an adequate and well-distributed intake of protein is vital. Plant-based sources of protein include legumes, tofu, tempeh, seitan, and a variety of nuts and seeds. Incorporating a combination of these sources throughout the day can help meet protein requirements and support overall health.

Carbohydrate Management: Carbohydrates directly impact blood sugar levels, making their management crucial for individuals with diabetes. While a vegan diet tends to be rich in carbohydrates from fruits, vegetables, and whole grains, the focus should be on complex carbohydrates with a low glycemic index. This includes quinoa, barley, sweet potatoes, and whole grain products. Distributing carbohydrate intake evenly across meals and snacks can help stabilize blood sugar levels.

Essential Fatty Acids: Omega-3 and omega-6 fatty acids are essential for cardiovascular health and overall well-being. Vegans can obtain these fatty acids from sources such as flaxseeds, chia seeds, walnuts, hemp seeds, and algae-based supplements. Balancing the intake of these fats contributes to a heart-healthy diet, which is particularly relevant for individuals with diabetes considering their increased risk of cardiovascular complications.

Vitamins and Minerals: Ensuring sufficient intake of essential vitamins and minerals is crucial for overall health, and this becomes even more pronounced for individuals with diabetes. Key nutrients include vitamin B12, vitamin D, iron, zinc, and calcium. Vegans should be vigilant in sourcing these nutrients from fortified foods or supplements when necessary, as some are primarily found in animal products.

Fiber-Rich Foods: Fiber plays a significant role in diabetes management by slowing down the absorption of glucose and promoting satiety. A vegan diet, rich in fruits, vegetables, whole grains, and legumes, naturally provides ample dietary fiber. Emphasizing a variety of fiber sources contributes to digestive health and supports glycemic control.

Hydration: Staying adequately hydrated is essential for everyone, but individuals with diabetes should pay particular attention to their fluid intake. Water is the best choice, and avoiding sugary beverages aligns with both diabetes management and overall health goals. Herbal teas and infused water can add variety to hydration options without adding unnecessary sugars.

Navigating these nutritional considerations requires a thoughtful and individualized approach. Consulting with a registered dietitian or nutritionist with expertise in plant-based nutrition and diabetes management is invaluable. These professionals can provide personalized guidance, ensuring that nutritional needs are met while supporting overall health and diabetes management.

Understanding the nuances of diabetes and its impact on individuals choosing a vegan lifestyle is essential for effective management. Recognizing the potential benefits, addressing nutritional concerns, and embracing a holistic approach to well-being can empower individuals to thrive in their journey with diabetes. As we move forward in this exploration, subsequent chapters will delve into the practical aspects of adopting a vegan lifestyle with diabetes, providing actionable insights for everyday life.

Chapter 2:

Building a Plant-Based Diabetes Management Plan

Living well with diabetes as a vegan involves more than just choosing plant-based foods; it requires a thoughtful and strategic approach to crafting a diabetes management plan. This chapter explores the power of plants in providing key nutrients for diabetes control, guides on crafting balanced vegan meals for effective blood sugar management, and insights into meal planning and portion control tailored to the needs of individuals with diabetes.

The Power of Plants: Key Nutrients for Diabetes Control

A plant-based diet offers a wealth of essential nutrients that play a pivotal role in diabetes control. Understanding and harnessing the power of these plant-derived elements is key to building an effective diabetes management plan.

Fiber: A Foundation for Blood Sugar Control

One of the standout features of a plant-based diet is its high fiber content. Fiber is a non-digestible carbohydrate that comes in two forms: soluble and insoluble. Soluble fiber, found in foods like oats, beans, and lentils, has been shown to slow down the absorption of glucose, preventing sudden spikes in blood sugar levels. Insoluble fiber, prevalent in whole grains and many vegetables, contributes to digestive health, aiding in weight management—a crucial aspect of diabetes control.

By emphasizing fiber-rich foods, individuals with diabetes can achieve better blood sugar control and maintain stable energy levels throughout the day. Including a variety of fruits, vegetables, whole grains, and legumes in daily meals ensures an ample supply of both types of fiber, contributing to overall well-being.

Antioxidants: Fighting Oxidative Stress

Plant-based foods are rich in antioxidants, compounds that help neutralize harmful free radicals in the body. Oxidative stress is implicated in the development of diabetes-related complications, making antioxidants particularly valuable for individuals with diabetes. Fruits and vegetables, especially those with vibrant colors like berries, spinach, and kale, are potent sources of antioxidants.

Including a diverse array of colorful plant foods in the diet not only enhances the visual appeal of meals but also provides a spectrum of antioxidants with different protective properties. This diversity helps combat oxidative stress, supporting the body's defense against diabetes-related complications.

Plant-Based Proteins: Nurturing Muscles and Metabolism

Protein is a crucial macronutrient for individuals with diabetes, playing a role in muscle maintenance, metabolic function, and satiety. Plant-based proteins, derived from sources like beans, lentils, tofu, and tempeh, offer a nutrient-dense and heart-healthy alternative to animal-based proteins.

Incorporating a variety of plant-based protein sources into meals ensures a comprehensive amino acid profile, supporting overall health. Additionally, these protein-rich foods contribute to a sense of fullness, assisting in weight management—an essential aspect of diabetes control.

Healthy Fats: Nourishing the Body and Brain

While individuals with diabetes need to be mindful of their fat intake, including healthy fats in the diet is crucial for overall health. Plant-based fats, such as those found in avocados, nuts, seeds, and olive oil, provide essential fatty acids that support brain function, reduce inflammation, and contribute to cardiovascular health.

Balancing the intake of healthy fats is essential for individuals with diabetes, and incorporating them into meals adds flavor and satiety. A well-rounded diabetes management plan includes these fats in moderation, contributing to a holistic approach to health.

Complex Carbohydrates: Sustained Energy for Diabetes Management

Carbohydrates are a primary source of energy, and the type of carbohydrates consumed can significantly impact blood sugar levels. Plant-based diets emphasize complex carbohydrates found in whole grains, vegetables, and legumes. These carbohydrates release glucose into the bloodstream more slowly, providing sustained energy and preventing rapid spikes in blood sugar.

Choosing whole, minimally processed plant foods over refined carbohydrates is a fundamental aspect of diabetes control. This approach ensures a steady supply of energy while supporting overall health through the wealth of nutrients found in these complex carbohydrate sources.

Understanding the power of these plant-derived nutrients and incorporating them into a well-balanced diet lays the foundation for effective diabetes control. The next section explores practical strategies for crafting balanced vegan meals that prioritize these key elements.

Crafting Balanced Vegan Meals for Blood Sugar Management

Creating balanced meals is a cornerstone of effective diabetes management for individuals following a vegan lifestyle. This section provides insights into building meals that prioritize key nutrients, support stable blood sugar levels, and contribute to overall well-being.

Balancing Macronutrients: The Plate Method

The plate method is a practical and visual approach to meal planning that helps individuals create well-balanced and portion-controlled meals. Dividing the plate into sections for different food groups—vegetables, grains, and proteins—encourages a thoughtful distribution of macronutrients.

For individuals with diabetes, the plate method is particularly useful in managing carbohydrate intake. By dedicating a portion of the plate to non-starchy vegetables, a quarter to lean proteins, and a quarter to whole grains or other complex carbohydrates, meals can be designed to support stable blood sugar levels. This method also facilitates portion control, a crucial aspect of diabetes management.

Emphasizing Non-Starchy Vegetables: Nutrient Density and Low Glycemic Impact

Non-starchy vegetables are a nutritional powerhouse for individuals with diabetes. Rich in fiber, vitamins, and minerals, these vegetables contribute to satiety without significantly impacting blood sugar levels. Including a variety of colorful vegetables such as leafy greens, broccoli, cauliflower, and bell peppers in each meal enhances the nutritional profile while adding vibrant flavors and textures.

The low glycemic impact of non-starchy vegetables makes them a valuable component of meals for individuals with diabetes. They provide essential nutrients without causing rapid spikes in blood sugar, contributing to effective glycemic control.

Choosing Whole Grains: Complex Carbohydrates for Sustained Energy

Whole grains are a staple in a balanced vegan diet, offering complex carbohydrates that release glucose gradually into the bloodstream. This sustained release of energy helps prevent sudden spikes in blood sugar levels, supporting stable glycemic control.

Including whole grains such as quinoa, brown rice, barley, and oats in meals provides not only carbohydrates but also essential nutrients like fiber, vitamins, and minerals. These nutrient-dense grains contribute to overall health while addressing the specific dietary needs of individuals with diabetes.

Plant-Based Proteins: A Foundation for Balanced Meals

Plant-based proteins are a key component of balanced vegan meals, providing essential amino acids and supporting muscle health. Incorporating a variety of protein sources, such as beans, lentils, tofu, and tempeh, ensures a comprehensive nutrient profile while contributing to satiety.

Balancing protein intake with other macronutrients helps create meals that promote fullness, prevent overeating, and support weight management—a critical aspect of diabetes control. Additionally, plant-based proteins often come with additional benefits, such as fiber and antioxidants, further enhancing the nutritional quality of meals.

Healthy Fats: Enhancing Flavor and Nutrient Absorption

Including healthy fats in meals not only adds flavor and texture but also enhances the absorption of fat-soluble vitamins. Plant-based fats from sources like avocados, nuts, seeds, and olive oil contribute to the overall nutritional quality of meals.

Balancing the intake of healthy fats supports cardiovascular health, a crucial consideration for individuals with diabetes who are at an increased risk of heart-related complications. Practicing moderation and incorporating a variety of plant-based fats into meals ensures a well-rounded approach to diabetes management.

Crafting balanced vegan meals involves thoughtful consideration of these components, creating a harmonious combination of nutrients that support blood sugar management and overall health. The following section delves into the practical aspects of meal planning and portion control tailored to the needs of individuals with diabetes.

Meal Planning and Portion Control for Vegans with Diabetes

Effective diabetes management for individuals following a vegan lifestyle requires intentional meal planning and portion control. This section provides practical strategies and insights into creating meal plans that align with dietary preferences, meet nutritional needs, and contribute to stable blood sugar levels.

Understanding Glycemic Index and Load

The glycemic index (GI) and glycemic load (GL) are tools that help individuals with diabetes make informed choices about the carbohydrates they consume. The GI measures how quickly a carbohydrate-containing food raises blood sugar, while the GL considers both the quality and quantity of carbohydrates in a serving.

Favoring low-GI and low-GL foods in meal planning can help individuals with diabetes manage their blood sugar levels effectively. Many plant-based foods, such as non-starchy vegetables, whole grains, and legumes, have a low glycemic impact, making them suitable choices for stable glycemic control.

Creating a Weekly Meal Plan

A weekly meal plan provides structure and helps individuals with diabetes make intentional choices about their food intake. Planning meals allows for a balanced distribution of macronutrients, ensures variety in food choices, and simplifies the grocery shopping process.

When crafting a weekly meal plan, individuals can incorporate a mix of plant-based proteins, whole grains, non-starchy vegetables, and healthy fats. This variety not only supports nutritional needs but also adds diversity to meals, making the overall eating experience more enjoyable.

Smart Snacking Strategies

Snacking can be a part of a well-balanced diabetes management plan, provided it is done mindfully. Opting for nutrient-dense snacks that include a combination of protein, fiber, and healthy fats can help prevent blood sugar spikes between meals.

Examples of smart snacks for individuals with diabetes include a handful of nuts, sliced vegetables with hummus, or a piece of fruit with nut butter. These options provide sustained energy and contribute to satiety without compromising blood sugar control.

Understanding Portion Control

Portion control is a crucial aspect of diabetes management, helping individuals regulate their calorie intake and maintain a healthy weight. While the specific portion sizes may vary based on individual needs and activity levels, adopting mindful eating practices can support overall well-being.

Using visual cues, such as the plate method mentioned earlier, or measuring portions with tools like measuring cups can assist individuals in managing their food intake. Being mindful of portion sizes, especially for carbohydrate-rich foods, helps prevent overeating and supports stable blood sugar levels.

Flexibility and Adaptability

While a structured meal plan provides guidance, it's essential to recognize the importance of flexibility and adaptability. Life is dynamic, and circumstances may arise that require adjustments to the plan. Being adaptable allows individuals to make informed choices in various situations, such as dining out, traveling, or unexpected schedule changes.

Flexibility also extends to accommodating personal preferences and tastes. A vegan diet offers a vast array of plant-based foods, allowing individuals to tailor their meal plans to align with their culinary preferences and cultural influences. Embracing this flexibility contributes to a positive and sustainable approach to diabetes management.

Building a plant-based diabetes management plan involves leveraging the power of plant-derived nutrients, crafting balanced meals, and implementing practical strategies for meal planning and portion control. By understanding the intricacies of these components, individuals with diabetes can create a sustainable and enjoyable approach to their dietary choices, supporting both their health and their commitment to a vegan lifestyle. As we delve further into this exploration, subsequent chapters will provide additional insights into smart shopping, cooking techniques, and navigating social situations as a vegan managing diabetes.

Chapter 3:

Vegan-Friendly Alternatives for Blood Sugar Control

As individuals with diabetes navigate the landscape of a vegan lifestyle, it's essential to explore alternatives that contribute to effective blood sugar control. This chapter delves into vegan-friendly options that specifically address this need, including plant-based sweeteners, low-glycemic index foods, and protein sources that sustain energy and promote a sense of fullness.

Plant-Based Sweeteners and Their Impact on Blood Glucose

The quest for sweetness in a diabetic-friendly, vegan diet often leads to the exploration of plant-based sweeteners. Understanding their impact on blood glucose levels is crucial for making informed choices that align with both dietary preferences and health goals.

Natural Sweeteners: A Healthier Indulgence

Natural sweeteners derived from plant sources offer a more wholesome alternative to refined sugars. Maple syrup, agave nectar, and date syrup are examples of sweeteners with distinctive flavors that can enhance the taste of various dishes. These natural options often contain additional nutrients such as vitamins and minerals, providing a nutritional boost along with sweetness.

While these sweeteners may be perceived as healthier choices, it's essential to use them in moderation. Even natural sugars can affect blood sugar levels, so individuals with diabetes should be mindful of portion sizes and overall carbohydrate intake.

Incorporating these sweeteners into a well-balanced meal, where the sugars are accompanied by fiber and other nutrients, can help mitigate their impact on blood glucose.

Stevia: A Zero-Calorie Sweet Solution

Stevia, a natural sweetener derived from the leaves of the Stevia rebaudiana plant, has gained popularity for its zero-calorie status and minimal impact on blood sugar levels. It is much sweeter than traditional sugar, requiring only a small amount to achieve the desired sweetness. This makes stevia a suitable option for those with diabetes looking to satisfy their sweet tooth without a significant impact on their glycemic profile.

When using stevia, it's crucial to choose high-quality, pure forms without added sugars or fillers. Experimenting with the amount to find the right balance in recipes allows individuals to enjoy sweetness without compromising their blood sugar control.

Monk Fruit: Nature's Sweet Secret

Monk fruit, also known as luo han guo, is another natural sweetener gaining attention for its unique sweetness derived from mogrosides. Similar to stevia, monk fruit is a zero-calorie sweetener that does not spike blood sugar levels. It is available in various forms, including liquid extracts and granulated sweeteners, making it a versatile choice for sweetening beverages, desserts, and other culinary creations.

As with any sweetener, moderation is key. Monk fruit can be an excellent addition to a vegan diet for individuals with diabetes, offering a sweet taste without the potential drawbacks associated with traditional sugars.

Coconut Sugar: A Low-Glycemic Sweet Option

Derived from the sap of coconut palm trees, coconut sugar is a natural sweetener with a lower glycemic index compared to traditional sugars. While it still contains carbohydrates and sugars, the presence of inulin—a type of fiber—may contribute to a slower rise in blood sugar levels.

Coconut sugar's caramel-like flavor makes it a popular choice in both sweet and savory dishes. However, like other sweeteners, it should be used in moderation. Including it as part of a well-balanced meal helps offset its impact on blood glucose levels.

Understanding the nuances of these plant-based sweeteners empowers individuals with diabetes to make choices that align with their health goals. Experimenting with different sweeteners, mindful portion control, and incorporating them into meals rich in fiber and nutrients contribute to a more diabetes-friendly approach to sweetness.

Exploring Low-Glycemic Index Foods for Vegans

The glycemic index (GI) is a valuable tool for individuals with diabetes, helping them choose foods that have a minimal impact on blood sugar levels. Exploring low-GI foods within a vegan framework offers a wide array of options that contribute to effective blood sugar control and overall well-being.

Legumes: Protein-Packed and Low-Glycemic

Legumes, including beans, lentils, and chickpeas, are staples in a vegan diet and offer a dual benefit for individuals with diabetes. Rich in plant-based protein and fiber, legumes have a low glycemic index, contributing to sustained energy and stable blood sugar levels.

The fiber content in legumes slows down the digestion and absorption of carbohydrates, preventing rapid spikes in blood glucose. Additionally, the protein content promotes a sense of fullness, making legumes an excellent choice for those looking to manage their weight alongside blood sugar levels.

Quinoa: A Complete Protein with Low Glycemic Impact

Quinoa stands out among grains for its status as a complete protein, providing all essential amino acids. Beyond its protein-rich profile, quinoa has a low glycemic index, making it a valuable addition to a diabetic-friendly, vegan diet.

The combination of protein and complex carbohydrates in quinoa supports sustained energy release, making it an excellent choice for meals that contribute to overall glycemic control. Whether used as a base for salads, a side dish, or a breakfast option, quinoa adds nutritional value and versatility to the vegan plate.

Nuts and Seeds: Healthy Fats and Low-GI Goodness

Nuts and seeds, including almonds, walnuts, chia seeds, and flaxseeds, are nutrient-dense foods with a low glycemic index. While they contain healthy fats, the fiber content helps mitigate their impact on blood sugar levels.

Incorporating nuts and seeds into meals and snacks adds crunch, flavor, and a wealth of essential nutrients. Whether sprinkled on salads, blended into smoothies, or enjoyed as a snack, these low-GI options contribute to a balanced and diabetes-friendly vegan diet.

Non-Starchy Vegetables: The Foundation of Low-GI Eating

Non-starchy vegetables are a cornerstone of a low-GI, vegan diet. With a vast array of options such as leafy greens, broccoli, cauliflower, and bell peppers, these vegetables are rich in fiber, vitamins, and minerals, providing essential nutrients without significantly affecting blood sugar levels.

The low glycemic impact of non-starchy vegetables makes them suitable for frequent inclusion in meals. Whether enjoyed raw, steamed, or roasted, these vegetables contribute to the overall nutritional quality of the vegan diet while supporting effective blood sugar control.

Berries: Antioxidant-rich and Low-Glycemic

Berries, including strawberries, blueberries, and raspberries, are not only rich in antioxidants but also have a low glycemic index. The natural sweetness of berries makes them a satisfying and diabetes-friendly option for adding sweetness to meals and snacks.

Berries can be enjoyed on their own, added to smoothies, or incorporated into desserts for a burst of flavor without causing significant fluctuations in blood sugar levels. Their versatility and nutritional benefits make them an excellent choice for individuals with diabetes following a vegan lifestyle.

Incorporating these low-GI foods into a vegan diet supports effective blood sugar control while providing a wealth of essential nutrients. Experimenting with different combinations and recipes allows individuals to enjoy a diverse and satisfying range of options that contribute to their overall health.

Vegan Protein Sources for Sustained Energy and Fullness

Protein is a crucial macronutrient for individuals with diabetes, contributing to satiety, muscle health, and overall well-being.

Exploring vegan protein sources that align with blood sugar control goals ensures sustained energy and a sense of fullness.

Lentils: Protein-Packed Legumes

Lentils are a versatile and protein-rich legume that deserves a prominent place in the vegan diet for individuals with diabetes. With a low glycemic index and high fiber content, lentils contribute to stable blood sugar levels while promoting satiety.

From lentil soups to salads and stews, the adaptability of lentils makes them a go-to protein source for vegan meals. The variety of lentil types, including brown, green, and red, offers different textures and flavors to suit various culinary preferences.

Tofu: A Versatile Plant-Based Protein

Tofu, made from soybeans, is a versatile and protein-rich option for individuals following a vegan diet. With a neutral flavor, tofu absorbs the tastes of the dishes it's incorporated into, making it suitable for savory and sweet preparations.

In addition to its protein content, tofu contains essential amino acids and is a good source of iron and calcium. Whether grilled, stir-fried, or blended into smoothies, tofu contributes to sustained energy and a feeling of fullness, making it a valuable component of a diabetes-friendly, vegan diet.

Chickpeas: Protein-Packed and Fiber-Rich

Chickpeas, also known as garbanzo beans, are a staple in vegan diets and offer a robust combination of protein and fiber. With a low glycemic index, chickpeas provide a steady release of energy, making them an excellent choice for individuals with diabetes.

From hummus to roasted chickpea snacks and chickpea salads, there are numerous ways to incorporate these legumes into meals. The versatility of chickpeas, coupled with their nutritional benefits, makes them a valuable protein source for those seeking to manage blood sugar levels through a vegan lifestyle.

Nuts and Seeds: Plant-Based Proteins with Healthy Fats

Nuts and seeds not only provide healthy fats but are also rich sources of plant-based proteins. Almonds, walnuts, chia seeds, and flaxseeds are examples of nutrient-dense options that contribute to sustained energy and a feeling of fullness.

While nuts and seeds should be consumed in moderation due to their calorie density, incorporating them into meals and snacks adds texture, flavor, and nutritional value. Whether sprinkled on salads, blended into smoothies, or enjoyed as a nut butter spread, these plant-based proteins contribute to a balanced and satisfying vegan diet.

Seitan: A High-Protein Meat Substitute

Seitan, also known as wheat gluten, is a protein-rich meat substitute commonly used in vegan and vegetarian diets. With a chewy texture and the ability to absorb flavors, seitan is a versatile ingredient for creating plant-based versions of traditionally meat-centric dishes.

While seitan is an excellent source of protein, individuals with gluten sensitivity or celiac disease should exercise caution, as it is made from wheat gluten. For those without gluten-related concerns, incorporating seitan into meals offers a substantial protein boost.

Understanding these vegan protein sources and their role in blood sugar control empowers individuals with diabetes to create meals that align with their health goals. The combination of protein, fiber, and healthy fats from these sources contributes to a balanced and satisfying vegan diet that supports overall well-being.

Exploring vegan-friendly alternatives for blood sugar control involves making informed choices about sweeteners, incorporating low-GI foods, and selecting plant-based proteins that sustain energy and promote a sense of fullness. By embracing the diversity of plant-based options and experimenting with different culinary creations, individuals with diabetes can navigate the intersection of a vegan lifestyle and effective blood sugar management. As we move forward in this exploration, subsequent chapters will delve into practical tips for grocery shopping, cooking techniques, and strategies for dining out while maintaining a vegan and diabetes-friendly approach.

Chapter 4:

Meal Planning

Meal planning is a cornerstone of successful diabetes management within a vegan lifestyle. This chapter explores the art of creating delicious and nutritious vegan meals, provides sample meal plans tailored to different dietary needs, and emphasizes the importance of incorporating variety for sustainable nutrition. By understanding the principles of meal planning, individuals can navigate the intersection of a vegan diet and diabetes management with creativity and intentionality.

Creating Delicious and Nutritious Vegan Meals

Crafting delicious and nutritious vegan meals requires a thoughtful approach that balances flavors, textures, and nutritional content. This section delves into key considerations for creating meals that are both enjoyable and supportive of diabetes management.

Balancing Macronutrients: The Foundation of Meal Planning

A well-balanced vegan meal incorporates a mix of macronutrients—carbohydrates, proteins, and fats. For individuals with diabetes, this balance is crucial for stabilizing blood sugar levels and supporting overall health.

1. **Carbohydrates**: Choose complex carbohydrates with a low glycemic index, such as whole grains, legumes, and non-starchy vegetables. These provide sustained energy without causing rapid spikes in blood sugar.

2. **Proteins**: Include plant-based proteins from sources like tofu, tempeh, legumes, nuts, and seeds. Protein

contributes to satiety, helps maintain muscle health, and supports overall well-being.

3. **Fats**: Opt for healthy fats from sources like avocados, nuts, seeds, and plant-based oils. These fats provide essential fatty acids and contribute to a satisfying and flavorful meal.

Colorful and Diverse Plates: Maximizing Nutrient Intake

A visually appealing plate often signifies a diverse and nutrient-rich meal. Aim to include a variety of colors, textures, and flavors in each meal to ensure a broad spectrum of essential nutrients.

1. **Vegetables**: Fill half your plate with a colorful array of non-starchy vegetables. These provide vitamins, minerals, and antioxidants while contributing to a feeling of fullness.

2. **Whole Grains**: Choose whole grains such as quinoa, brown rice, or barley as a base for your meals. These grains offer complex carbohydrates, fiber, and additional nutrients.

3. **Proteins**: Incorporate plant-based proteins from a mix of sources to ensure a diverse amino acid profile. Rotate between tofu, tempeh, legumes, and other protein-rich foods to keep meals exciting.

4. **Healthy Fats**: Add a moderate amount of healthy fats to your meals for flavor and satiety. Avocado slices, a sprinkle of nuts or seeds, or a drizzle of olive oil can enhance both taste and nutrition.

Mindful Portion Control: Supporting Blood Sugar Management

Portion control is a key aspect of diabetes management, ensuring a balanced intake of calories and macronutrients. While individual needs may vary, adopting mindful eating practices can support overall well-being.

1. **Plate Method**: Use the plate method as a visual guide for portion control. Divide your plate into sections for non-starchy vegetables, whole grains, and plant-based proteins, with a side of healthy fats.

2. **Listening to Hunger Cues**: Pay attention to hunger and fullness cues. Eating slowly, savoring each bite, and stopping when satisfied contribute to a healthier relationship with food.

3. **Smart Snacking**: If snacking is part of your routine, choose nutrient-dense options like fresh fruit with nut butter, vegetable sticks with hummus, or a small handful of nuts. Snacking mindfully can prevent overconsumption.

Flavorful Cooking Techniques: Enhancing Culinary Enjoyment

Experimenting with different cooking techniques adds depth and flavor to vegan meals. While minimizing the use of added sugars and unhealthy fats, explore methods that bring out the natural tastes of ingredients.

1. **Roasting**: Roasting vegetables enhances their natural sweetness and creates a delightful caramelization. Toss your favorite veggies with a bit of olive oil and seasoning, then roast until golden and tender.

2. **Grilling**: Grilling adds a smoky flavor to plant-based proteins like tofu, tempeh, and vegetables. Marinate

ingredients in flavorful herbs and spices before grilling for an extra burst of taste.

3. **Sautéing**: Sautéing allows for quick and flavorful cooking. Use minimal oil and incorporate aromatic ingredients like garlic, ginger, or herbs to elevate the taste of your dishes.

4. **Steaming**: Steaming preserves the nutritional content of vegetables while providing a tender texture. Steam a variety of colorful vegetables for a vibrant and healthful side dish.

By embracing these principles, individuals can create vegan meals that are not only delicious but also supportive of diabetes management. The combination of mindful portion control, a variety of nutrient-dense foods, and flavorful cooking techniques contribute to a positive and enjoyable culinary experience.

Sample Meal Plans for Different Dietary Needs

Creating a meal plan tailored to individual dietary needs is essential for effective diabetes management. This section provides sample meal plans that cater to different preferences and requirements within the context of a vegan lifestyle.

Meal Plan 1: Balanced and Nutrient-Rich

Breakfast:

- **Quinoa Breakfast Bowl**

    - Cooked quinoa

    - Mixed berries

    - Chopped nuts (almonds or walnuts)

- Drizzle of maple syrup

- Plant-based milk

Lunch:

- **Chickpea and Vegetable Salad**

  - Chickpeas, cherry tomatoes, cucumber, red onion, and bell peppers

  - Fresh herbs (parsley or cilantro)

  - Olive oil and lemon dressing

  - Quinoa or brown rice on the side

Dinner:

- **Grilled** Tofu Stir-Fry

  - Tofu cubes marinated in soy sauce, ginger, and garlic

  - Stir-fried with a variety of colorful vegetables (broccoli, bell peppers, snap peas)

  - Brown rice or cauliflower rice

Snack:

- Sliced apple with almond butter

This balanced meal plan incorporates a mix of whole grains, plant-based proteins, and colorful vegetables to provide a range of essential nutrients while supporting blood sugar control.

Meal Plan 2: Quick and Convenient

Breakfast:

- **Smoothie Bowl**

  - Frozen berries

  - Banana

  - Spinach

  - Plant-based protein powder

  - Almond milk

  - Toppings: granola, chia seeds, and sliced almonds

Lunch:

- **Lentil Soup (canned or pre-made)**

  - Mixed green salad with a simple vinaigrette

  - Whole-grain roll or slice of whole-grain bread

Dinner:

- **Vegan Stir-Fried Noodles**

  - Buckwheat or rice noodles

  - Tofu or tempeh

  - Mixed vegetables (bell peppers, broccoli, carrots)

  - Soy sauce and sesame oil for flavor

Snack:

- **Hummus with carrot and cucumber sticks**

This meal plan is designed for convenience, incorporating quick and easy-to-prepare options while maintaining a balance of nutrients for sustained energy.

Meal Plan 3: High-Protein and Satiating

Breakfast:

- **Overnight Chia Pudding**
    - Chia seeds soaked in almond milk
    - Topped with sliced strawberries and a sprinkle of hemp seeds

Lunch:

- **Quinoa and Black Bean Bowl**
    - Quinoa
    - Black beans
    - Avocado slices
    - Salsa
    - Lime wedges

Dinner:

- **Baked Falafel with Mediterranean Salad**
    - Homemade or store-bought falafel
    - Mixed greens, cherry tomatoes, cucumber, olives
    - Tahini dressing

Snack:

- Roasted chickpeas

This high-protein meal plan prioritizes plant-based protein sources to support muscle health and provide a satisfying and satiating eating experience.

These sample meal plans serve as inspiration, illustrating the versatility and variety achievable within a vegan and diabetes-friendly diet. However, individual dietary needs and preferences vary, and it's essential to tailor meal plans to specific requirements.

Incorporating Variety for Sustainable Nutrition

Variety is a key principle in maintaining a sustainable and enjoyable vegan diet while managing diabetes. This section explores the importance of incorporating a diverse range of foods for both nutritional and culinary benefits.

Diverse Nutrient Intake: Maximizing Health Benefits

Consuming a variety of plant-based foods ensures a diverse intake of nutrients, promoting overall health and well-being. Each food group contributes unique vitamins, minerals, and antioxidants, supporting various bodily functions.

1. **Leafy Greens**: Incorporate a variety of leafy greens such as kale, spinach, collard greens, and Swiss chard. These greens are rich in vitamins A and K, folate, and iron.

2. **Colorful Vegetables**: Consume a spectrum of colorful vegetables to benefit from a range of antioxidants. Bell peppers, tomatoes, carrots, and eggplants each bring unique nutritional advantages to the table.

3. **Whole Grains**: Experiment with different whole grains to diversify your nutrient intake. Quinoa, barley, farro,

and bulgur provide distinct textures and nutritional profiles.

4. **Legumes**: Rotate between different legumes like lentils, chickpeas, black beans, and edamame. Each legume offers a unique combination of protein, fiber, and essential nutrients.

5. **Nuts and Seeds**: Include a variety of nuts and seeds in your diet for healthy fats, protein, and micronutrients. Almonds, walnuts, chia seeds, and flaxseeds contribute to a well-rounded nutritional profile.

6. **Fruits**: Explore a diverse selection of fruits to meet your vitamin and fiber needs. Berries, citrus fruits, apples, and bananas offer a mix of flavors and nutritional benefits.

7. **Plant-Based Proteins**: Incorporate a range of plant-based proteins to ensure a variety of amino acids. Tofu, tempeh, seitan, and legumes each bring unique textures and flavors to your meals.

Culinary Exploration: Enhancing Enjoyment

Incorporating variety into your meals is not only beneficial for nutrition but also enhances the enjoyment of your culinary experience. Culinary exploration allows for the discovery of new flavors, textures, and cultural influences.

1. **Global Cuisine Exploration**: Experiment with recipes from various cuisines around the world. Whether it's Mediterranean, Asian, Latin American, or Middle Eastern, each cuisine offers a rich tapestry of plant-based options.

2. **Seasonal Eating**: Embrace seasonal produce to enjoy fresh and flavorful ingredients at their peak. Seasonal eating adds natural variety to your meals and supports local and sustainable food choices.

3. **Herbs and Spices**: Elevate your dishes with a diverse array of herbs and spices. Cilantro, basil, turmeric, cumin, and paprika can transform the same ingredients into unique and exciting meals.

4. **Plant-Based Alternatives**: Explore the growing variety of plant-based alternatives in the market. From plant-based cheeses to meat substitutes, these options can add novelty and convenience to your meals.

Adaptability and Flexibility: Sustainable Lifestyle Choices

Maintaining a sustainable vegan lifestyle while managing diabetes involves adaptability and flexibility. Being open to trying new foods, recipes, and cooking techniques allows for a dynamic and enjoyable approach to plant-based living.

1. **Seasonal Meal Rotation**: Rotate your meals based on seasons and availability. This not only ensures a diverse nutrient intake but also keeps your meals interesting and aligned with what's fresh and abundant.

2. **Recipe Modification**: Modify and adapt recipes to suit your taste preferences and dietary needs. Experimenting with ingredient substitutions and cooking methods allows you to personalize meals while maintaining nutritional integrity.

3. **Mindful Eating Practices**: Practice mindful eating to fully appreciate the flavors and textures of each meal. Being present during meals promotes a positive

relationship with food and enhances the overall dining experience.

4. **Social and Cultural Influences**: Embrace social and cultural influences when it comes to food. Participate in potlucks, cooking classes, or food-related events to broaden your culinary horizons and connect with a community that shares your values.

Incorporating variety into your vegan and diabetes-friendly lifestyle is not only about nutritional benefits but also about fostering a sustainable and enjoyable relationship with food. By embracing a diverse range of plant-based foods and culinary influences, individuals can create meals that are both nourishing and exciting.

Meal planning within the context of a vegan lifestyle and diabetes management involves creating delicious and nutritious meals, tailoring sample meal plans to different dietary needs, and incorporating variety for sustainable nutrition. By approaching meal planning with creativity, intentionality, and an openness to culinary exploration, individuals can navigate the complexities of managing diabetes while enjoying the diverse and vibrant world of plant-based eating. As we progress in this exploration, subsequent chapters will delve into practical tips for cooking techniques, strategies for dining out, and further insights into optimizing a vegan and diabetes-friendly approach to nutrition.

Chapter 5:

Smart Shopping and Pantry Essentials

Effective diabetes management as a vegan begins with smart shopping and a well-stocked pantry. This chapter guides individuals through navigating the grocery store for diabetes-friendly vegan options, offers insights into stocking a pantry for success, and emphasizes the importance of reading food labels effectively to make informed choices aligned with health goals.

Navigating the Grocery Store for Diabetes-Friendly Vegan Options

Grocery shopping is a fundamental aspect of adopting a diabetes-friendly vegan lifestyle. Navigating the aisles with intentionality and awareness ensures that individuals make choices that support blood sugar control while adhering to their commitment to a plant-based diet.

Prioritizing Fresh Produce: The Foundation of a Vegan Diet

The produce section is a treasure trove of nutrient-dense foods that form the foundation of a diabetes-friendly vegan diet. Fresh fruits and vegetables, rich in fiber, vitamins, and minerals, contribute to overall well-being and support glycemic control.

When shopping for fresh produce, it's beneficial to include a variety of colors and types. Berries, leafy greens, cruciferous vegetables, and colorful peppers are excellent choices. Aim to include a diverse range of options in your cart to ensure a broad spectrum of nutrients that complement your health goals.

Choosing Whole Grains and Legumes: A Diabetes-Friendly Duo

Whole grains and legumes are valuable staples for individuals with diabetes following a vegan diet. These nutrient-dense foods provide complex carbohydrates, fiber, and plant-based proteins that contribute to sustained energy and stable blood sugar levels.

When selecting whole grains, options like quinoa, brown rice, oats, and whole wheat products are preferable. Legumes, including beans, lentils, and chickpeas, offer versatility and nutritional benefits. Opt for canned or dried legumes and whole grains to keep your pantry well-stocked for various culinary creations.

Exploring the Plant-Based Protein Aisle: Beyond Tofu and Tempeh

The plant-based protein aisle is expanding, offering an array of options beyond traditional tofu and tempeh. Explore plant-based protein alternatives like seitan, plant-based burgers, and meat substitutes made from ingredients like mushrooms and legumes.

While incorporating these options into your diet, it's essential to check the nutritional content and ingredient list. Some processed plant-based protein products may contain added sugars or unhealthy fats. Prioritize products with minimal additives and opt for those rich in protein and essential nutrients.

Navigating the Frozen Section: Convenience without Compromise

The frozen section of the grocery store provides convenient options for individuals with diabetes following a vegan lifestyle. Frozen fruits and vegetables, without added sauces or sugars, are excellent choices for quick and easy meal preparation.

In addition to produce, explore the frozen section for vegan-friendly frozen meals, veggie burgers, and plant-based protein alternatives. Pay attention to nutritional labels, focusing on products that align with your dietary and blood sugar management goals.

Choosing Healthy Fats: Oils, Nuts, and Seeds

Healthy fats play a crucial role in a balanced vegan diet, contributing to satiety and overall well-being. When navigating the grocery store, choose plant-based oils like olive oil, avocado oil, or flaxseed oil for cooking and salad dressings.

Nuts and seeds are essential pantry staples, providing healthy fats, protein, and an array of vitamins and minerals. Opt for unsalted and raw varieties to avoid added sodium and unnecessary processing. Including a variety of nuts and seeds in your diet ensures a diverse nutrient profile.

Be Mindful of Processed Vegan Foods: Moderation is Key

While the plant-based movement has led to an increase in vegan convenience foods, it's crucial to approach these products with moderation. Processed vegan foods, such as vegan cookies, snacks, and ready-to-eat meals, may contain added sugars, unhealthy fats, and preservatives.

When exploring these options, read labels carefully and prioritize whole, minimally processed foods. Incorporate processed vegan items as occasional treats rather than regular staples in your diet. This approach supports both blood sugar control and overall health.

Navigating the grocery store for diabetes-friendly vegan options involves a balance between fresh produce, whole grains, plant-based proteins, healthy fats, and mindful choices in the processed food aisle. By approaching shopping with intentionality and awareness, individuals can create a well-rounded and satisfying vegan diet that aligns with their health goals.

Stocking Your Pantry for Success

A well-stocked pantry is the backbone of a successful diabetes-friendly vegan kitchen. Stocking essential ingredients ensures that individuals have the tools and options needed for nutritious and delicious meals. This section explores key pantry essentials for those managing diabetes while adhering to a vegan lifestyle.

Whole Grains: The Foundation of a Nutrient-Dense Diet

Whole grains are a vital component of a diabetes-friendly vegan diet, providing complex carbohydrates, fiber, and essential nutrients. Stocking your pantry with a variety of whole grains ensures versatility in meal preparation.

Quinoa, brown rice, oats, barley, and whole wheat products are excellent choices. These whole grains serve as the base for hearty salads, grain bowls, and side dishes, contributing to sustained energy and stable blood sugar levels.

Legumes: Plant-Based Protein Powerhouses

Dried and canned legumes are pantry essentials for individuals following a vegan diet. Beans, lentils, and chickpeas are rich sources of plant-based protein, fiber, and an array of vitamins and minerals.

Having both dried and canned options allows for flexibility in meal planning. Canned legumes provide convenience for quick meals, while dried legumes offer a cost-effective and versatile alternative. Rinse canned legumes before use to reduce sodium content.

Nuts and Seeds: Versatile and Nutrient-Dense

Nuts and seeds are pantry staples that add texture, flavor, and nutritional value to meals. Almonds, walnuts, chia seeds, flaxseeds, and sunflower seeds are excellent choices.

Keep a variety of nuts and seeds on hand for snacking, adding to salads, or incorporating into recipes. These nutrient-dense foods contribute healthy fats, protein, and essential micronutrients to a well-balanced vegan diet.

Plant-Based Proteins: Diversify Your Options

In addition to legumes, diversify your plant-based protein sources by stocking your pantry with alternative protein options. Tofu, tempeh, and seitan are versatile choices that can be used in a variety of recipes.

Explore the plant-based protein aisle for vegan burgers, sausages, and other meat alternatives. Choose products with minimal additives and prioritize those rich in protein and essential nutrients.

Healthy Fats: Oils and Avocados

Healthy fats are crucial for overall health and satiety. Stock your pantry with plant-based oils such as olive oil, avocado oil, and flaxseed oil for cooking and salad dressings.

Avocados are a nutrient-dense source of healthy fats and can be kept on hand for adding creaminess to dishes or enjoyed on their own. Be mindful of portion sizes, as healthy fats are calorie-dense.

Whole-Food Sweeteners: Moderation in Sweetness

For those with a sweet tooth, having whole-food sweeteners in the pantry allows for the creation of delicious treats without compromising blood sugar control. Options such as maple syrup, agave nectar, and date syrup can add sweetness to recipes.

However, it's essential to use these sweeteners in moderation. When incorporating them into recipes, be mindful of overall carbohydrate intake and consider pairing sweeteners with fiber-rich ingredients for a balanced approach.

Canned Tomatoes and Tomato Products: A Kitchen Staple

Canned tomatoes and tomato products are versatile ingredients that can serve as a base for sauces, soups, stews, and more. Opt for varieties without added sugars or excessive sodium.

Tomatoes are rich in vitamins, minerals, and antioxidants, providing both flavor and nutritional value to a variety of dishes. Keeping these pantry staples ensures the ability to whip up quick and nutritious meals.

Herbs and Spices: Flavor Without Compromise

Herbs and spices are essential for creating flavorful dishes without relying on excessive salt, sugar, or unhealthy fats. Stock your pantry with a variety of herbs and spices, including basil, oregano, thyme, cumin, turmeric, and garlic powder.

Experimenting with different seasonings allows you to add complexity and depth to your meals. Herbs and spices not only enhance the taste of dishes but also contribute additional health benefits.

Whole-Grain Pasta and Rice Alternatives: Diverse Options

Explore the variety of whole-grain pasta and rice alternatives available in the market. Options such as brown rice pasta, quinoa pasta, and cauliflower rice provide alternatives with lower glycemic impact and higher nutritional value.

These alternatives can be used in place of traditional refined grains, contributing to better blood sugar control and overall health. Keep a selection on hand for diverse meal options.

By stocking your pantry with these essentials, you create a foundation for diabetes-friendly vegan meals that are both nutritious and satisfying. A well-prepared pantry ensures that you have the ingredients needed for diverse and flavorful dishes, supporting your commitment to a healthy and plant-based lifestyle.

Reading Food Labels Effectively

Reading food labels is a skill that empowers individuals to make informed choices about the products they consume. For those managing diabetes while adhering to a vegan lifestyle, understanding how to interpret food labels is particularly crucial. This section guides reading food labels effectively to support blood sugar control and overall health.

Serving Size: The Foundation of Nutritional Information

The serving size listed on a food label serves as the baseline for all nutritional information provided. Understanding the serving size is essential for accurately assessing the nutritional content of the product.

Pay attention to portion sizes and consider whether they align with your dietary goals. For individuals with diabetes, being mindful of carbohydrate intake is especially important, making the serving size a key factor in making informed choices.

Total Carbohydrates: Focus on Quality

Total carbohydrates on a food label encompass all types of carbohydrates, including sugars, fiber, and starches. For individuals with diabetes, focusing on the quality of carbohydrates is crucial for blood sugar control.

Prioritize foods that are rich in fiber and have a lower glycemic index. High-fiber foods, such as whole grains, legumes, and non-starchy vegetables, contribute to sustained energy and prevent rapid spikes in blood sugar levels.

Dietary Fiber: A Crucial Component

Dietary fiber is a nutrient that plays a significant role in diabetes management. It slows down the digestion and absorption of carbohydrates, promoting stable blood sugar levels and contributing to a feeling of fullness.

Look for products with higher dietary fiber content, as they provide additional health benefits. Foods rich in fiber are often more nutrient-dense and support overall digestive health.

Sugars: Distinguish Between Natural and Added

The sugars listed on a food label can come from natural sources, such as fruits and dairy, or be added during processing. Distinguishing between natural and added sugars is essential for those managing diabetes.

While natural sugars are part of whole foods and come with accompanying fiber and nutrients, added sugars can contribute to blood sugar spikes. Be cautious of products with high amounts of added sugars, and opt for those with minimal or no added sugars.

Protein: Prioritize Plant-Based Sources

Protein is a crucial macronutrient for individuals following a vegan diet, providing essential amino acids and supporting overall health. When reading food labels, prioritize products that are rich in plant-based proteins.

Look for sources like tofu, tempeh, legumes, nuts, and seeds. These plant-based protein options contribute to satiety and support muscle health, both important considerations for those managing diabetes.

Fats: Choose Healthy Fats in Moderation

While total fat content is listed on food labels, it's essential to distinguish between different types of fats. Choose products with healthy fats, such as monounsaturated and polyunsaturated fats, and limit saturated and trans fats.

Opt for plant-based oils, avocados, nuts, and seeds as sources of healthy fats. Be mindful of portion sizes, as fats are calorie-dense, and moderation is key for overall health.

Sodium: Monitor Sodium Intake

Sodium, or salt, is an ingredient that can impact blood pressure and overall cardiovascular health. Individuals with diabetes may be at an increased risk of heart-related complications, making it important to monitor sodium intake.

Choose products with lower sodium content, especially when using canned or processed foods. Rinsing canned legumes and vegetables can help reduce sodium levels.

Ingredient List: Understand What Goes into Your Food

The ingredient list on a food label provides valuable insights into the composition of a product. Ingredients are listed in descending order by weight, with the primary ingredient listed first.

Be mindful of added sugars, unhealthy fats, and preservatives in the ingredient list. Opt for products with recognizable and whole-food ingredients, and be cautious of overly processed items.

Allergen Information: Ensure Dietary Compatibility

For individuals with allergies or dietary restrictions, checking allergen information is crucial. Food labels typically include information about common allergens, such as nuts, soy, and gluten.

Ensure that the product aligns with your dietary preferences and any specific restrictions you may have. Cross-check allergen information to avoid unintended consumption of allergens.

Certifications: Look for Vegan and Diabetes-Friendly Labels

Certifications on food labels can provide additional reassurance regarding a product's suitability for a vegan and diabetes-friendly lifestyle. Look for certifications such as "vegan," which ensures the absence of animal-derived ingredients, and labels indicating suitability for individuals with diabetes.

Certifications from reputable organizations can simplify the decision-making process and offer peace of mind when selecting products.

Reading food labels effectively is a skill that becomes increasingly valuable when managing diabetes on a vegan diet.

By understanding the nuances of nutritional information, individuals can make choices that align with their health goals and dietary preferences. This skill empowers individuals to navigate the grocery store with confidence and select products that contribute to overall well-being.

The combination of smart shopping, well-stocked pantry essentials, and effective reading of food labels forms the basis for successful diabetes management within a vegan lifestyle. By approaching these aspects with intentionality, individuals can create a sustainable and enjoyable approach to their dietary choices, supporting both their health and commitment to a vegan way of life. As we proceed in this exploration, subsequent chapters will provide insights into practical cooking techniques, meal planning, and strategies for dining out within the context of a vegan and diabetes-friendly lifestyle.

Chapter 6:

Cooking Techniques and Tips

Cooking techniques play a pivotal role in the success of a vegan and diabetes-friendly lifestyle. This chapter delves into healthy cooking methods, explores how to add flavorful seasonings without compromising health, and provides quick and easy cooking hacks for individuals with busy lifestyles. By mastering these techniques, individuals can create delicious and nutritious meals that align with their dietary goals.

Healthy Cooking Methods

Choosing the right cooking methods can significantly impact the nutritional content of your meals. This section explores healthy cooking methods that preserve the integrity of plant-based ingredients, support blood sugar management, and contribute to overall well-being.

1. *Steaming: Preserving Nutrients and Texture*

Steaming is a gentle cooking method that helps retain the nutritional content of vegetables while maintaining their natural textures. This technique involves cooking food over boiling water, allowing steam to circulate and cook the ingredients.

When steaming vegetables, aim for vibrant colors and a crisp-tender texture. Vegetables such as broccoli, carrots, cauliflower, and green beans steam beautifully. This method is particularly beneficial for those managing diabetes, as it avoids the need for added fats and oils.

2. *Grilling: Adding Flavor Without Excess Fats*

Grilling is a popular cooking method that imparts a smoky flavor to plant-based proteins and vegetables. This technique involves cooking food over an open flame or hot surface, typically on a grill or grill pan.

For a diabetes-friendly approach, marinate tofu, tempeh, or vegetables in flavorful, low-sugar marinades before grilling. The high heat caramelizes the surfaces, enhancing the taste without the need for excessive oils. Grilling is a versatile method that can add variety to your meals, especially during warmer seasons.

3. *Baking and Roasting: Enhancing Natural Flavors*

Baking and roasting are dry heat cooking methods that can enhance the natural flavors of ingredients. These methods involve cooking food in an oven at high temperatures.

When baking or roasting, use parchment paper or non-stick cooking spray to minimize the need for added fats. This technique is particularly useful for preparing dishes like roasted vegetables, baked tofu, or even whole-grain casseroles. The dry heat can intensify flavors and create appealing textures.

4. *Sautéing: Quick and Flavorful Cooking*

Sautéing is a quick and versatile cooking method that involves cooking food rapidly in a small amount of oil over medium-high heat. It's an excellent way to cook a variety of vegetables, tofu, and legumes.

For a diabetes-friendly approach, use heart-healthy oils like olive oil and control the amount used. Combine colorful vegetables with tofu or beans for a quick and nutritious sauté. Experimenting with different herbs and spices can elevate the flavors without compromising health.

5. *Slow Cooking: Simplicity and Flavor Fusion*

Slow cooking, or using a crockpot, is a convenient method that allows ingredients to simmer and meld flavors over an extended period. This technique is ideal for busy individuals as it requires minimal hands-on time.

When slow cooking, opt for whole, minimally processed ingredients. This method works well for dishes like vegetable stews, bean soups, or lentil-based curries. Slow cooking allows for a depth of flavor development without the need for excessive fats or sugars.

6. *Boiling: Retaining Nutrients in Liquids*

Boiling involves cooking food in water at its boiling point. While it may seem like a simple method, boiling can be a healthy option, especially when preparing soups, stews, or grains.

To retain the nutrients in the cooking liquid, consider using vegetable broth or water infused with herbs and spices. Boiling is an effective way to cook grains like quinoa or brown rice without adding extra fats, supporting a diabetes-friendly approach.

Healthy cooking methods prioritize the preservation of nutrients and the reduction of unnecessary fats. By incorporating these techniques into your culinary repertoire, you can create flavorful and nutritious meals that align with both a vegan lifestyle and diabetes management.

Flavorful Seasonings Without Compromising Health

Seasonings are the heart of flavorful cooking, but it's essential to choose options that align with a diabetes-friendly and vegan lifestyle. This section explores ways to add depth and taste to your dishes without compromising health.

1. *Herbs and Spices: Nature's Flavor Enhancers*

Herbs and spices are potent flavor enhancers that bring depth and complexity to dishes without the need for added sugars or unhealthy fats. Experimenting with a variety of herbs and spices allows you to create diverse and exciting flavor profiles.

1. **Basil:** Fresh or dried basil adds a sweet, slightly peppery flavor to dishes. It pairs well with tomatoes, making it an excellent addition to pasta sauces, salads, and Mediterranean-inspired dishes.

2. **Cumin:** Cumin offers a warm, earthy flavor with a hint of citrus. It's a versatile spice that complements legumes, grains, and roasted vegetables. Use cumin to add depth to chili, curries, or roasted chickpeas.

3. **Turmeric:** Known for its vibrant yellow color, turmeric has a warm, slightly bitter taste. It's a staple in many curry blends and pairs well with lentils, rice, and roasted cauliflower. Turmeric also offers anti-inflammatory properties.

4. **Thyme:** With a subtle, earthy flavor, thyme is a versatile herb that works well in soups, stews, and roasted dishes. It pairs beautifully with lentils, mushrooms, and root vegetables.

5. **Oregano:** Oregano has a robust and slightly peppery flavor. It's a classic herb in Mediterranean cuisine and adds a delightful touch to tomato-based sauces, roasted vegetables, and homemade pizza.

6. **Paprika:** Paprika comes in various types, each with its flavor profile—sweet, smoked, or hot. It's a colorful

addition to dishes like soups, stews, and roasted potatoes.

7. **Cilantro:** Cilantro, also known as coriander leaves, adds a fresh and citrusy flavor to dishes. It's a key ingredient in many Mexican, Thai, and Indian recipes, providing a burst of brightness.

2. Citrus Zest and Juices: Brightening Flavors Naturally

Citrus fruits, such as lemons, limes, and oranges, offer a natural way to brighten and enhance flavors. Using citrus zest and juices in your cooking adds acidity and freshness without the need for excess salt or sugars.

1. **Lemon Zest:** Grated lemon zest adds a burst of citrusy aroma and flavor. Use it in dressings, marinades, or as a finishing touch on roasted vegetables or grains.

2. **Lime Juice:** Lime juice brings a tangy and slightly sweet element to dishes. It pairs well with cilantro in Mexican-inspired dishes, adds brightness to stir-fries, and elevates the flavor of fruit salads.

3. **Orange Zest:** Orange zest contributes a sweet and aromatic essence to both sweet and savory dishes. Incorporate it into marinades for tofu, sauces, or desserts for a citrusy twist.

3. Vinegar: Enhancing Flavors with Acidity

Vinegar, both traditional and infused varieties, provides acidity that enhances and balances flavors in a wide range of dishes.

1. **Balsamic Vinegar:** Balsamic vinegar adds a rich, sweet, and tangy flavor. It's an excellent choice for drizzling

over roasted vegetables and salads or using it as a glaze for tofu or tempeh.

2. **Apple Cider Vinegar:** With a slightly fruity and tangy taste, apple cider vinegar works well in dressings, marinades, and pickling liquids. It can add a refreshing element to slaws or grain salads.

3. **Rice Vinegar:** Rice vinegar offers a milder acidity and is commonly used in Asian cuisines. It's suitable for making sushi rice, light salad dressings, or pickling vegetables.

4. *Nutritional Yeast: Umami and Cheesy Flavor*

Nutritional yeast is a vegan pantry staple known for its umami-rich and slightly cheesy flavor. It's often used to add depth to plant-based dishes.

1. **Sprinkle on Popcorn:** Nutritional yeast can be sprinkled on popcorn for a savory and cheesy twist. It's a guilt-free alternative to traditional cheese flavorings.

2. **In Vegan Cheeses:** Use nutritional yeast as a base for homemade vegan cheeses. It adds a cheesy flavor to cashew or almond-based cheese sauces.

3. **In Pasta Dishes:** Stir nutritional yeast into pasta sauces for a creamy and cheesy element. It pairs well with tomato-based or Alfredo-style sauces.

5. *Homemade Spice Blends: Customizing Flavors*

Creating your spice blends allows you to customize flavors to suit your preferences while avoiding added sugars, sodium, or preservatives.

1. **Curry Powder:** Blend cumin, coriander, turmeric, and other spices for a homemade curry powder. Use it to season lentil dishes, soups, or roasted vegetables.

2. **Italian Seasoning:** Mix dried basil, oregano, thyme, rosemary, and garlic powder for an Italian seasoning blend. Sprinkle it on pasta, pizza, or roasted dishes.

3. **Taco Seasoning:** Combine chili powder, cumin, paprika, garlic powder, and onion powder for a homemade taco seasoning. Use it to season tofu, beans, or plant-based meat alternatives.

By incorporating these flavorful seasonings into your cooking, you can create vibrant and enticing dishes without compromising your commitment to a vegan and diabetes-friendly lifestyle.

Quick and Easy Cooking Hacks for Busy Lifestyles

For individuals with busy lifestyles, efficient and practical cooking hacks can make a significant difference. This section explores quick and easy cooking tips that streamline meal preparation while maintaining the health-conscious approach of a vegan and diabetes-friendly lifestyle.

1. Batch Cooking and Meal Prep: Streamlining the Week

Batch cooking and meal prep are invaluable techniques for individuals with hectic schedules. Devote a specific time during the week to prepare and cook large quantities of staple ingredients.

1. **Cooking Grains:** Prepare a large batch of quinoa, brown rice, or other whole grains to use throughout the week. Portion them into containers for quick and convenient access.

2. **Chopping Vegetables:** Wash, peel, and chop a variety of vegetables in advance. Having pre-cut veggies on hand accelerates the cooking process and encourages the inclusion of colorful and nutrient-rich options.

3. **Marinating Proteins:** Marinate tofu, tempeh, or plant-based proteins in bulk. Store them in the refrigerator or freezer, ready to be quickly grilled, baked, or sautéed for a protein-packed meal.

2. *One-Pot and Sheet Pan Meals: Simplifying Cleanup*

Streamline both cooking and cleanup with one-pot and sheet pan meals. These techniques involve cooking an entire meal in a single pot or on a single sheet pan.

1. **One-Pot Pasta:** Combine pasta, vegetables, plant-based proteins, and a flavorful sauce in one pot. The ingredients cook together, infusing the pasta with rich flavors and reducing the number of dishes to clean.

2. **Sheet Pan Roasting:** Toss vegetables, tofu, or tempeh with your favorite herbs and spices on a sheet pan. Roast them in the oven for an easy, hands-off meal that requires minimal cleanup.

3. **Stir-Fry: Quick and Flavorful Cooking:** Stir-frying is a rapid cooking method that involves tossing ingredients in a pan over high heat. Use a variety of colorful vegetables, tofu, and a simple sauce for a speedy and delicious meal.

3. *Frozen Fruits and Vegetables: Convenience Without Compromise*

While fresh produce is ideal, frozen fruits and vegetables offer convenience without sacrificing nutritional quality. They are pre-washed, and pre-cut, and often retain their nutritional value.

1. **Smoothie Packs:** Create smoothie packs by portioning out frozen fruits, greens, and any additional ingredients. Store these packs in the freezer for quick and effortless smoothie preparation.

2. **Stir-Fry Staples:** Keep a variety of frozen vegetables on hand for quick stir-fries. They can be added directly to the pan, eliminating the need for chopping and reducing cooking time.

3. **Frozen Berries for Oatmeal:** Add frozen berries directly to oatmeal during cooking. They provide natural sweetness and a burst of antioxidants without the need for added sugars.

4. *Instant Pot and Pressure Cooking: Speedy Cooking Solutions*

The Instant Pot and other pressure cookers are valuable tools for accelerating cooking times while preserving the nutritional content of ingredients.

1. **Beans and Legumes:** Use the Instant Pot to cook dried beans and legumes quickly. This method eliminates the need for pre-soaking and significantly reduces cooking time.

2. **Whole Grains:** Pressure cookers efficiently prepare whole grains like brown rice, quinoa, and farro. This allows for quick meal assembly without compromising the nutritional benefits of whole grains.

3. **Soups and Stews:** Create flavorful soups and stews in a fraction of the time with pressure cooking. Combine a variety of vegetables, plant-based proteins, and spices for a hearty and efficient meal.

5. *Pre-Packaged Salad Mixes: Effortless Greens*

Pre-packaged salad mixes offer a convenient way to incorporate greens into your meals without the need for extensive washing and chopping.

1. **Quick Salad Bases:** Choose pre-packaged salad mixes as a base for quick salads. Add additional fresh vegetables, nuts, seeds, and a simple dressing for a nutritious and hassle-free meal.

2. **Stir-Fry Enhancements:** Use pre-packaged stir-fry mixes as a foundation for quick and colorful stir-fries. Simply add tofu, tempeh, or plant-based proteins for a complete and speedy meal.

3. **Smoothie Boosts:** Many stores offer pre-packaged smoothie mixes with a variety of fruits and greens. These can be combined with plant-based milk for a quick and nutrient-packed smoothie.

Incorporating these quick and easy cooking hacks into your routine allows for efficient meal preparation without compromising the health-conscious approach of a vegan and diabetes-friendly lifestyle. By simplifying the cooking process, individuals with busy lifestyles can continue to enjoy delicious and nutritious meals while managing their dietary needs effectively.

Mastering healthy cooking methods, choosing flavorful seasonings without compromising health, and adopting quick and easy cooking hacks are essential components of a successful vegan and diabetes-friendly lifestyle. By incorporating these techniques into your culinary repertoire, you can create a diverse range of meals that are not only delicious but also supportive of your health goals. As we progress in this exploration, subsequent chapters will provide insights into dining out, managing special occasions, and further optimizing a plant-based approach to diabetes management.

Chapter 7:

Eating Out and Social Situations

Eating out and navigating social situations can present unique challenges for individuals following a vegan and diabetes-friendly lifestyle. This chapter explores strategies for making wise choices at restaurants, offers insights into navigating social gatherings and celebrations, and emphasizes effective communication of dietary needs. By mastering these aspects, individuals can maintain their commitment to health and ethical choices while enjoying the social aspects of dining.

Making Wise Choices at Restaurants

Choosing to dine out doesn't mean compromising your commitment to a vegan and diabetes-friendly lifestyle. With careful consideration and awareness, you can make wise choices at restaurants that align with your dietary preferences and health goals.

1. *Researching Restaurant Menus in Advance*

Before heading to a restaurant, take advantage of online resources to research their menu. Many establishments now provide their menus on their websites or through apps. Look for vegan and plant-based options, and consider the ingredients used in different dishes.

1. **Vegan-Friendly Restaurants:** Choose restaurants known for their vegan-friendly options. These establishments are more likely to have a variety of plant-based choices, making it easier to find a meal that aligns with both your vegan and diabetes-friendly requirements.

2. **Customization Options:** Check if the restaurant allows customization of dishes. Many places are willing to accommodate dietary preferences, such as substituting certain ingredients or adjusting cooking methods.

3. **Nutritional Information:** Some restaurants provide nutritional information for their dishes. Look for information on carbohydrate content, fiber, and overall calorie count, which can be particularly helpful for managing diabetes.

2. Choosing Whole, Minimally Processed Foods

Opting for whole, minimally processed foods is a key principle in both vegan and diabetes-friendly diets. When scanning the menu, focus on dishes that feature whole plant-based ingredients.

1. **Whole Grains:** Choose dishes that incorporate whole grains such as quinoa, brown rice, or barley. These grains offer fiber and nutrients that contribute to stable blood sugar levels.

2. **Vegetable-Centric Options:** Look for dishes that are rich in vegetables. Non-starchy vegetables are low in carbohydrates and high in fiber, making them an excellent choice for individuals managing diabetes.

3. **Plant-Based Proteins:** Select dishes that include plant-based proteins like tofu, tempeh, legumes, or seitan. These proteins provide essential amino acids without the saturated fats found in some animal products.

3. Being Mindful of Cooking Methods

The way a dish is prepared can significantly impact its nutritional content. Be mindful of cooking methods, and choose options that align with both a vegan lifestyle and diabetes management.

1. **Grilled or Roasted:** Opt for dishes that are grilled or roasted, as these methods often require minimal added fats. Grilled vegetables, tofu, or plant-based proteins can be flavorful and satisfying.

2. **Steamed or Sautéed:** Choose dishes that are steamed or sautéed with minimal oil. These methods preserve the natural flavors of ingredients while minimizing the need for added fats.

3. **Avoiding Fried Options:** Limit fried and deep-fried choices, as these cooking methods can introduce excess unhealthy fats and impact blood sugar levels. If possible, ask if items can be prepared using alternative cooking methods.

4. *Controlling Portion Sizes*

Portion control is crucial for managing diabetes, and many restaurants tend to serve larger portions. Take steps to control portion sizes to avoid overeating and better manage blood sugar levels.

1. **Sharing Dishes:** Consider sharing dishes with dining companions. This allows you to enjoy a variety of flavors without consuming excessive portions.

2. **Ordering Half Portions:** Inquire if the restaurant offers half portions or the option to customize the size of your dish. This can be particularly helpful in managing carbohydrate intake.

3. **Taking Home Leftovers:** If the portions are generous, don't hesitate to ask for a takeout container. Taking leftovers home not only prevents overeating but also provides a delicious meal for the next day.

By approaching restaurant dining with awareness and a strategic mindset, individuals can enjoy the experience while staying true to their vegan and diabetes-friendly lifestyle.

Navigating Social Gatherings and Celebrations

Social gatherings and celebrations often revolve around food, and navigating these situations requires thoughtful planning to maintain your commitment to a vegan and diabetes-friendly lifestyle. The following strategies can help you navigate social events with confidence.

1. Communication with Hosts in Advance

If possible, communicate with the event hosts in advance to discuss your dietary preferences and any specific dietary needs related to diabetes. This proactive approach allows hosts to accommodate your requirements and ensures that you'll have suitable options available.

1. **Expressing Gratitude:** Begin the conversation by expressing gratitude for the invitation and enthusiasm for attending the event. Emphasize that you're looking forward to the gathering and appreciate their efforts in hosting.

2. **Clarifying Dietary Needs:** Communicate your dietary needs related to both veganism and diabetes. Mention any specific ingredients to avoid or include, and politely ask if there's an opportunity to collaborate on the menu.

3. **Offering to Contribute:** If appropriate, offer to bring a dish to share. This ensures there will be at least one option that aligns with your dietary preferences and allows you to contribute to the communal aspect of the gathering.

2. Scanning the Menu or Buffet Strategically

When faced with a buffet or a variety of food options, approach the situation strategically to make choices that align with your vegan and diabetes-friendly lifestyle.

1. **Surveying Options:** Before diving in, take a moment to survey all the food options available. This allows you to make informed decisions based on the variety of dishes.

2. **Prioritizing Whole Foods:** Focus on whole, minimally processed foods. Look for vegetable-centric options, whole grains, and plant-based proteins to create a balanced and satisfying plate.

3. **Mindful Portion Control:** Be mindful of portion sizes, especially if the event offers a buffet or a variety of dishes. Start with smaller portions, and go back for more if needed, ensuring better control over your overall carbohydrate intake.

3. Strategizing Alcohol Consumption

Alcohol can impact blood sugar levels, and many social gatherings involve drinks. Consider these strategies to manage alcohol consumption while staying true to your diabetes-friendly lifestyle.

1. **Choosing Low-Sugar Options:** Opt for low-sugar or sugar-free drink options. Selecting dry wines, light

beers, or spirits with sugar-free mixers can help minimize the impact on blood sugar levels.

2. **Alternate with Water:** Alternate alcoholic beverages with water. This not only helps control your overall alcohol intake but also keeps you hydrated throughout the event.

3. **Setting Limits:** Establish personal limits for alcohol consumption and stick to them. Knowing your boundaries ensures that you can enjoy the social aspect of the gathering without compromising your health goals.

4. *Handling Questions and Comments Gracefully*

In social settings, you may encounter questions or comments about your dietary choices. Handling these situations with grace and confidence is essential.

1. **Educating Politely:** If someone expresses curiosity about your vegan or diabetes-friendly choices, respond politely and informatively. Educate them on the health benefits and ethical considerations that guide your dietary decisions.

2. **Focusing on Positivity:** Emphasize the positive aspects of your dietary choices rather than dwelling on restrictions. Share the delicious and diverse foods you enjoy, and highlight how your choices contribute to your overall well-being.

3. **Redirecting Conversations:** If you find yourself in a situation where dietary choices become a focal point, gracefully redirect the conversation to other shared interests or topics. This allows you to enjoy the social

gathering without undue focus on your dietary preferences.

By employing these strategies, individuals can confidently navigate social gatherings and celebrations, fostering a positive and inclusive atmosphere while adhering to their vegan and diabetes-friendly lifestyle.

Communicating Your Dietary Needs Effectively

Effective communication is paramount when it comes to ensuring that your dietary needs are met, especially in social settings. This section explores strategies for communicating your vegan and diabetes-friendly requirements clearly and assertively.

1. *Expressing Dietary Needs Clearly*

When communicating your dietary needs, clarity is key. Clearly express your requirements related to both veganism and diabetes management, ensuring that there is a mutual understanding between you and those responsible for meal preparation.

1. **Using Direct Language:** Be direct and specific when communicating your dietary needs. Clearly state that you follow a vegan lifestyle and specify any dietary restrictions related to diabetes, such as limiting added sugars or controlling carbohydrate intake.

2. **Providing Examples:** Offer examples of foods that align with your dietary preferences. This can help others better understand the types of dishes or ingredients that are suitable for your vegan and diabetes-friendly lifestyle.

3. **Emphasizing Health Goals:** Communicate that your dietary choices are motivated by health goals and ethical considerations. This helps others appreciate the importance of your choices and may foster a supportive and understanding environment.

2. Collaborating on Meal Planning

If appropriate, collaborate with hosts or event organizers on meal planning. This collaboration ensures that there are options available that align with your dietary preferences and diabetes management.

1. **Offering Suggestions:** Provide suggestions for dishes that are both vegan and suitable for diabetes management. This collaborative approach helps hosts by offering concrete ideas for accommodating your needs.

2. **Sharing Recipes:** If comfortable, share vegan and diabetes-friendly recipes that hosts can consider incorporating into the menu. This not only provides practical solutions but also allows you to contribute to the culinary diversity of the event.

3. **Confirming Ingredients:** Before the event, confirm the ingredients used in certain dishes to ensure they align with your dietary requirements. This proactive step minimizes the risk of encountering unexpected ingredients.

3. Handling Dietary Preferences Diplomatically

In social situations, it's crucial to handle dietary preferences diplomatically to maintain positive interactions and a harmonious atmosphere.

1. **Expressing Gratitude for Efforts:** Regardless of the outcome, express gratitude for any efforts made to accommodate your dietary needs. Acknowledge the thoughtfulness and consideration shown by hosts or organizers.

2. **Being Flexible and Understanding:** Be flexible and understanding if certain accommodations cannot be met. In some situations, factors such as limited resources or culinary expertise may impact the ability to provide specific dishes.

3. **Offering to Contribute:** If feasible, offer to contribute a dish or share the responsibility for meal preparation. This collaborative approach demonstrates your commitment to the gathering while ensuring that your dietary needs are met.

Effective communication is a cornerstone of successfully navigating social situations while adhering to a vegan and diabetes-friendly lifestyle. By expressing your needs clearly, collaborating on meal planning when possible, and handling dietary preferences diplomatically, you can enjoy social gatherings while maintaining your commitment to health and ethical choices.

Mastering the art of making wise choices at restaurants, navigating social gatherings and celebrations, and effectively communicating dietary needs are essential aspects of maintaining a vegan and diabetes-friendly lifestyle. By approaching these situations with mindfulness, preparation, and positive communication, individuals can enjoy the social aspects of dining while staying true to their health and ethical principles. As we continue our exploration, subsequent chapters will provide insights into optimizing nutrition for specific situations, addressing common challenges, and further enhancing the overall well-being of individuals following a vegan and diabetes-friendly lifestyle.

Chapter 8:

Exercise and Physical Activity for Vegans with Diabetes

Physical activity is a cornerstone of diabetes management, and when combined with a vegan lifestyle, it becomes a powerful tool for overall health and well-being. This chapter explores the pivotal role of exercise in diabetes management for vegans, provides insights into tailoring exercise routines to support blood sugar control, and discusses the benefits of combining cardiovascular and strength training within a vegan framework.

The Role of Exercise in Diabetes Management for Vegans

Exercise is a crucial component of diabetes management for individuals following a vegan lifestyle. It offers a range of benefits that contribute to better blood sugar control, increased insulin sensitivity, and improved overall health.

1. *Enhancing Insulin Sensitivity*

Regular exercise has a profound impact on insulin sensitivity, a key factor in managing diabetes. Insulin sensitivity refers to how effectively the body's cells respond to insulin, the hormone responsible for regulating blood sugar levels.

1. **Muscle Glucose Uptake:** During exercise, muscles contract and increase their demand for glucose as a source of energy. This process enhances the ability of muscle cells to take up glucose from the bloodstream, reducing blood sugar levels.

2. **Improved Insulin Function:** Exercise helps improve the function of insulin in the body. As individuals engage in physical activity, insulin becomes more effective at

facilitating the uptake of glucose by cells, promoting better blood sugar regulation.

3. **Reduced Insulin Resistance:** Regular exercise reduces insulin resistance, a condition where cells become less responsive to insulin. Lowering insulin resistance is particularly beneficial for individuals with diabetes, as it improves the body's ability to utilize insulin for glucose uptake.

2. Weight Management and Metabolic Health

Maintaining a healthy weight is essential for diabetes management, and exercise plays a pivotal role in achieving and sustaining weight goals.

1. **Caloric Expenditure:** Exercise contributes to caloric expenditure, helping individuals achieve a calorie deficit if weight loss is a goal. This is vital for managing body weight and preventing excess fat accumulation.

2. **Muscle Mass Preservation:** Strength training exercises, in particular, help preserve and build lean muscle mass. This is crucial for individuals with diabetes, as muscle tissue plays a significant role in glucose metabolism.

3. **Enhanced Metabolic Rate:** Regular physical activity increases metabolic rate, even during periods of rest. This means that individuals who engage in consistent exercise burn more calories throughout the day, supporting weight management.

3. Blood Sugar Regulation and Long-Term Health Benefits

Exercise has immediate and long-term effects on blood sugar regulation, contributing to better overall health for individuals with diabetes.

1. **Post-Exercise Glucose Uptake:** The benefits of exercise extend beyond the duration of the activity. Following exercise, muscles continue to take up glucose, leading to improved post-exercise blood sugar levels.

2. **Cardiovascular Health:** Regular physical activity supports cardiovascular health, reducing the risk of heart disease, a common concern for individuals with diabetes. Cardiovascular exercise enhances circulation, lowers blood pressure, and improves lipid profiles.

3. **Stress Reduction:** Exercise has stress-reducing effects, which can be particularly beneficial for individuals managing diabetes. Chronic stress can impact blood sugar levels, and incorporating exercise into a routine helps mitigate stress and its potential impact on diabetes management.

4. **Improved Sleep:** Quality sleep is essential for overall health, including blood sugar regulation. Regular exercise promotes better sleep patterns, contributing to enhanced diabetes management.

In summary, the role of exercise in diabetes management for vegans is multifaceted. It positively influences insulin sensitivity, supports weight management, and offers both immediate and long-term benefits for blood sugar control and overall health.

Creating an exercise routine tailored to support blood sugar control is essential for individuals with diabetes following a vegan lifestyle. By considering the type, intensity, and timing of exercise, individuals can optimize the impact of physical activity on their diabetes management.

1. *Choosing Appropriate Exercise Types*

Different types of exercise have varying effects on blood sugar levels. When tailoring an exercise routine for blood sugar control, it's crucial to incorporate a combination of aerobic, strength training, and flexibility exercises.

1. **Aerobic Exercise:** Also known as cardiovascular exercise, aerobic activities like walking, jogging, cycling, and swimming have a direct impact on lowering blood sugar levels. Aim for at least 150 minutes of moderate-intensity aerobic exercise per week, spread across most days.

2. **Strength Training:** Incorporating strength training exercises at least two days a week is beneficial for blood sugar control. These exercises, which can include weightlifting, bodyweight exercises, or resistance band workouts, contribute to increased insulin sensitivity.

3. **Flexibility and Balance:** Activities such as yoga or tai chi enhance flexibility and balance. While they may not have a direct impact on blood sugar levels, they contribute to overall well-being and can be valuable components of an exercise routine.

2. *Monitoring Blood Sugar Levels During Exercise*

Monitoring blood sugar levels before, during, and after exercise is crucial for understanding how physical activity affects individual responses. This monitoring allows for adjustments to be made in real time to prevent hypoglycemia (low blood sugar) or hyperglycemia (high blood sugar).

1. **Pre-Exercise Checks:** Check blood sugar levels before starting any exercise, especially if using insulin or certain medications. This baseline measurement provides information on current blood sugar status.

2. **During Exercise Checks:** For longer or more intense workouts, consider checking blood sugar levels periodically. This is particularly important for individuals prone to hypoglycemia, ensuring that adjustments can be made if needed.

3. **Post-Exercise Checks:** Monitoring blood sugar levels after exercise helps individuals understand how their bodies respond to different activities. It also provides insights into the duration of post-exercise effects on blood sugar levels.

3. Balancing Nutrition and Exercise

Nutrition plays a crucial role in supporting blood sugar control during and after exercise. Consider these strategies for balancing nutrition with physical activity:

1. **Pre-Exercise Snacks:** Consume a small, balanced snack before exercising to provide a source of easily digestible carbohydrates. This helps prevent hypoglycemia during the workout.

2. **Hydration:** Staying hydrated is essential for overall health and can support blood sugar regulation. Drink

water before, during, and after exercise to maintain proper hydration.

3. **Post-Exercise Nutrition:** Consuming a balanced meal or snack after exercise helps replenish glycogen stores and supports recovery. Include a combination of carbohydrates, protein, and healthy fats.

4. **Timing Meals and Medications:** Consider the timing of meals and medications concerning the exercise routine. Adjustments may be necessary to prevent fluctuations in blood sugar levels.

4. Setting Realistic Goals and Gradual Progression

When tailoring an exercise routine, setting realistic goals and progressing gradually are key to long-term success. Individuals should consider their current fitness level, any existing health conditions, and the need for gradual adaptation.

1. **Starting Slow:** Begin with activities of low to moderate intensity, especially if new to regular exercise. This allows the body to adapt and minimizes the risk of injury or adverse reactions.

2. **Incremental Progression:** Gradually increase the duration, intensity, and frequency of exercise over time. This incremental progression helps the body adapt and minimizes the risk of overtraining or burnout.

3. **Setting Achievable Goals:** Establish achievable short-term and long-term goals. Celebrate small victories along the way, whether it's completing a certain duration of exercise or achieving a specific fitness milestone.

By tailoring exercise routines to support blood sugar control, individuals with diabetes following a vegan lifestyle can maximize the benefits of physical activity while minimizing potential challenges.

Combining Cardiovascular and Strength Training as a Vegan

A well-rounded exercise routine for individuals with diabetes following a vegan lifestyle should include a combination of cardiovascular and strength training exercises. This synergy provides comprehensive benefits for blood sugar control, cardiovascular health, and overall fitness.

1. *Cardiovascular Exercise for Blood Sugar Control*

Cardiovascular exercise, also known as aerobic exercise, is instrumental in blood sugar control for individuals with diabetes. The following considerations highlight the role of cardiovascular exercise within a vegan framework:

1. **Type of Cardiovascular Exercise:** Choose activities that you enjoy and can sustain over time. Options include walking, running, cycling, swimming, dancing, or participating in aerobic classes. The key is to engage in activities that elevate the heart rate and promote cardiovascular health.

2. **Frequency and Duration:** Aim for at least 150 minutes of moderate-intensity aerobic exercise per week, as recommended by health guidelines. This can be achieved through daily or weekly sessions, depending on individual preferences and schedules.

3. **Interval Training:** Consider incorporating interval training, alternating between periods of higher intensity

and lower intensity. Interval training has been shown to improve insulin sensitivity and enhance cardiovascular fitness.

4. **Vegan-Friendly Cardio Options:** Many cardiovascular exercises align seamlessly with a vegan lifestyle. For example, running, cycling, and swimming are inherently vegan, and options like dance or aerobics can be tailored to vegan preferences.

2. Strength Training for Insulin Sensitivity

Strength training, also known as resistance training or weightlifting, is a valuable complement to cardiovascular exercise for individuals with diabetes. It contributes to increased insulin sensitivity, improved muscle mass, and enhanced metabolic function.

1. **Type of Strength Training:** Incorporate a variety of strength training exercises that target different muscle groups. This can include bodyweight exercises, free weights, resistance bands, or machines. Choose exercises that align with personal preferences and any existing health considerations.

2. **Frequency and Progression:** Aim for strength training sessions at least two days per week, allowing for sufficient rest between sessions. Gradually increase the intensity, repetitions, or resistance over time to promote continuous progression.

3. **Full-Body Workouts:** Consider full-body workouts that engage multiple muscle groups simultaneously. This approach maximizes the efficiency of strength training sessions and promotes overall functional fitness.

4. **Vegan Protein Sources for Recovery:** After strength training, prioritize post-workout nutrition to support recovery. Vegan protein sources such as legumes, tofu, tempeh, and plant-based protein supplements can contribute to muscle repair and growth.

3. *Balancing Cardiovascular and Strength Training*

Combining cardiovascular and strength training exercises within a vegan framework provides a comprehensive approach to diabetes management and overall well-being. Consider the following strategies for balancing these two types of exercise:

1. **Creating a Balanced Routine:** Design an exercise routine that includes both cardiovascular and strength training elements. This balance ensures that different aspects of physical fitness are addressed, contributing to overall health.

2. **Alternating Workout Days:** Structure workout days to alternate between cardiovascular and strength training. This allows specific muscle groups to recover while engaging in complementary forms of exercise.

3. **Incorporating Flexibility and Recovery:** Include flexibility exercises, such as yoga or stretching, to enhance overall flexibility and support recovery. These activities can be integrated on rest days or as part of a well-rounded workout routine.

4. **Listening to Your Body:** Pay attention to your body's signals and adjust the balance of cardiovascular and strength training based on individual responses, energy levels, and recovery needs.

4. *Vegan Nutrition to Support Exercise*

Optimizing nutrition is crucial when engaging in a combination of cardiovascular and strength training exercises. For individuals following a vegan lifestyle, considerations for nutrient intake become paramount:

1. **Adequate Protein Intake:** Ensure sufficient protein intake to support muscle repair and growth. Include a variety of plant-based protein sources in your diet, such as legumes, lentils, tofu, tempeh, quinoa, and plant-based protein supplements if needed.

2. **Balanced Carbohydrates:** Maintain a balanced intake of carbohydrates to provide energy for both cardiovascular and strength training exercises. Choose whole, complex carbohydrates such as whole grains, fruits, and vegetables.

3. **Healthy Fats:** Include sources of healthy fats, such as avocados, nuts, seeds, and olive oil, to support overall health and provide a source of sustained energy.

4. **Hydration:** Stay well-hydrated before, during, and after exercise. Water is essential for optimal performance, recovery, and overall health.

5. **Supplementation if Necessary:** Consider supplementing with vitamin B12, vitamin D, and omega-3 fatty acids, which are nutrients that may require special attention in a vegan diet.

Combining cardiovascular and strength training within a vegan framework offers a holistic approach to diabetes management and overall health. Tailoring exercise routines to support blood sugar control, monitoring blood sugar levels, balancing nutrition, setting realistic goals, and embracing a well-rounded approach contribute to a successful and sustainable exercise regimen for individuals with diabetes following a vegan lifestyle. As we delve further into this exploration, subsequent chapters will address additional aspects of living well with diabetes as a vegan, including optimizing nutrition for specific situations, overcoming challenges, and thriving in the long term.

Chapter 9:

Navigating Vegan Challenges and Diabetes Complications

Living with diabetes on a vegan diet requires thoughtful consideration and strategic planning. This chapter delves into the potential nutritional deficiencies associated with vegan diets, offers insights into managing diabetes complications within a plant-based lifestyle, and explores vegan-friendly strategies for foot and eye care.

Vegan Diets and Potential Nutritional Deficiencies

While a well-planned vegan diet can provide all the nutrients the body needs, there are certain considerations to ensure optimal nutrition, especially for individuals managing diabetes. Understanding potential nutritional deficiencies and adopting proactive measures can help maintain a balanced and healthful vegan lifestyle.

1. *Vitamin B12 and Plant-Based Sources*

Vitamin B12 is essential for nerve function, red blood cell production, and the metabolism of nutrients. As it is primarily found in animal products, vegans need to pay special attention to ensuring adequate B12 intake.

1. **Plant-Based Sources:** While plant-based foods do not naturally contain vitamin B12, fortified foods and supplements are vegan-friendly options. Fortified plant milk, breakfast cereals, and nutritional yeast are common sources. Supplements, either B12-only or in multivitamins, are also widely available.

2. **Supplementation Guidelines:** Vegans, particularly those with diabetes, may benefit from regular B12 supplementation. It's advisable to consult with a healthcare professional to determine the appropriate dosage based on individual needs and potential interactions with diabetes medications.

3. **Regular Monitoring:** Periodic monitoring of B12 levels through blood tests is recommended to ensure sufficiency. This is especially important for individuals with diabetes, as vitamin B12 deficiency can exacerbate neurological complications associated with diabetes.

2. *Iron and Absorption Enhancers*

Iron is vital for transporting oxygen in the blood, and its absorption can be influenced by dietary factors. Plant-based sources of iron are abundant but are non-heme iron, which is not as easily absorbed as heme iron found in animal products.

1. **Iron-rich plant Foods:** Include iron-rich plant foods in the diet, such as lentils, beans, tofu, nuts, seeds, and dark leafy greens. Consuming vitamin C-rich foods alongside iron-rich meals can enhance non-heme iron absorption.

2. **Avoiding Inhibitors:** Limit the consumption of iron absorption inhibitors, such as tea and coffee, during meals. These beverages contain compounds that can hinder the absorption of non-heme iron.

3. **Cooking in Cast Iron:** Cooking in cast iron pans can contribute to dietary iron intake. The iron leaches into the food, providing an additional source of this essential mineral.

3. *Calcium and Bone Health*

Calcium is crucial for bone health, and individuals on a vegan diet need to ensure an adequate intake, particularly if they have diabetes, as bone health can be compromised by diabetes-related complications.

1. **Plant-Based Calcium Sources:** Incorporate plant-based calcium sources like fortified plant milk, tofu, kale, broccoli, and almonds into the diet. Choose fortified foods to meet calcium requirements.

2. **Calcium-Rich Supplements:** If necessary, calcium supplements can be considered. Ensure that the chosen supplement is vegan-friendly and consult with a healthcare professional for guidance on dosage.

3. **Vitamin D Synthesis:** Exposure to sunlight stimulates the synthesis of vitamin D in the skin. Ensure safe sun exposure to support vitamin D production, especially in regions with limited sunlight. Consider vitamin D supplementation if needed.

4. *Omega-3 Fatty Acids and Algal Oil*

Omega-3 fatty acids play a crucial role in heart and brain health. While fatty fish is a traditional source of these essential fats, vegans can obtain them from plant-based sources and algal oil supplements.

1. **Plant-Based Omega-3 Sources:** Include flaxseeds, chia seeds, hemp seeds, walnuts, and algae in the diet. Algal oil, derived from algae, provides a direct source of both EPA and DHA, the two primary forms of omega-3s.

2. **Supplementation Considerations:** Omega-3 supplementation with algal oil can be a convenient and effective option for ensuring adequate intake. As with any supplementation, consultation with a healthcare provider is advisable.

3. **Balancing Omega-3 and Omega-6 Ratio:** While omega-3s are important, maintaining a balanced ratio with omega-6 fatty acids is also crucial. Limiting the intake of processed oils rich in omega-6s can help maintain this balance.

By proactively addressing potential nutritional deficiencies, individuals following a vegan diet, especially those with diabetes, can ensure comprehensive and well-rounded nutrition.

Managing Diabetes Complications in a Plant-Based Lifestyle

Individuals with diabetes, regardless of their dietary choices, may face complications that require careful management. In a plant-based lifestyle, addressing these complications involves a combination of dietary choices, lifestyle modifications, and regular healthcare monitoring.

1. *Blood Sugar Management for Cardiovascular Health*

Cardiovascular health is a significant concern for individuals with diabetes, and a plant-based lifestyle offers unique advantages in managing both blood sugar levels and cardiovascular risk factors.

1. **Whole Food Plant-Based Diet:** Emphasize a whole food plant-based diet, rich in fruits, vegetables, whole grains, legumes, and nuts. This dietary approach is naturally

low in saturated fats and cholesterol, supporting heart health.

2. **Fiber-rich foods:** Prioritize fiber-rich foods to aid in blood sugar control and promote cardiovascular health. Foods like oats, beans, lentils, and vegetables contribute to satiety and assist in managing weight.

3. **Healthy Fats:** Choose sources of healthy fats, such as avocados, nuts, seeds, and olive oil, in moderation. These fats can contribute to cardiovascular health without compromising blood sugar control.

2. *Managing Hypertension and Kidney Health*

Hypertension and kidney complications are common concerns for individuals with diabetes. A plant-based lifestyle can contribute to managing these conditions through dietary choices and lifestyle modifications.

1. **Sodium Awareness:** Monitor sodium intake, as excessive sodium can contribute to hypertension. Choose whole, minimally processed foods and limit the use of added salt during cooking and at the table.

2. **Potassium-rich foods:** Include potassium-rich foods, such as bananas, oranges, potatoes, and leafy greens, to support blood pressure regulation. Potassium helps balance the effects of sodium in the body.

3. **Adequate Hydration:** Maintain adequate hydration to support kidney health. Water is essential for kidney function, and proper hydration can help prevent complications associated with dehydration.

3. *Neuropathy and Nerve Health*

Diabetes-related neuropathy can impact nerve function, leading to pain, tingling, and numbness. A plant-based lifestyle can contribute to nerve health through specific dietary choices and lifestyle practices.

1. **B-Vitamin-Rich Foods:** Incorporate foods rich in B vitamins, such as lentils, beans, leafy greens, and fortified foods. B vitamins are crucial for nerve health and can support individuals with neuropathy.

2. **Anti-Inflammatory Diet:** Adopt an anti-inflammatory diet by including foods with anti-inflammatory properties, such as berries, turmeric, ginger, and green leafy vegetables. Chronic inflammation can contribute to nerve damage.

3. **Blood Sugar Control:** Maintaining optimal blood sugar control is paramount in preventing and managing neuropathy. Consistent monitoring, medication adherence, and lifestyle modifications contribute to this effort.

4. Eye Health and Plant-Based Nutrition

Diabetes can affect eye health, leading to conditions such as diabetic retinopathy. A plant-based lifestyle can support eye health through specific nutrients and antioxidants.

1. **Lutein and Zeaxanthin-Rich Foods:** Include foods rich in lutein and zeaxanthin, such as kale, spinach, collard greens, and broccoli. These antioxidants contribute to eye health and may help prevent macular degeneration.

2. **Vitamin A Sources:** Consume foods rich in vitamin A, like sweet potatoes, carrots, and butternut squash.

Vitamin A is essential for maintaining the health of the retina and preventing night blindness.

3. **Omega-3 Fatty Acids:** Ensure an adequate intake of omega-3 fatty acids, found in algal oil, flaxseeds, chia seeds, and walnuts. Omega-3s support overall eye health and may reduce the risk of certain eye conditions.

By adopting a plant-based lifestyle and making mindful dietary choices, individuals with diabetes can actively contribute to the prevention and management of complications associated with the condition.

Vegan-Friendly Strategies for Foot and Eye Care

Foot and eye care are integral aspects of managing diabetes, and individuals on a vegan diet can leverage specific strategies to address these concerns effectively.

1. *Foot Care and Neuropathy Prevention*

Diabetes-related neuropathy can affect the feet, making proper foot care essential for preventing complications. Vegan-friendly strategies focus on maintaining foot health through attentive practices.

1. **Regular Foot Inspections:** Conduct regular foot inspections to identify any changes, injuries, or abnormalities. This proactive approach allows for early intervention and prevents complications.

2. **Moisturization:** Keep the feet well-moisturized to prevent dry skin and cracking. Choose vegan-friendly, non-irritating moisturizers to maintain skin health.

3. **Proper Footwear:** Wear comfortable and supportive shoes to reduce the risk of injuries and pressure points. Vegan-friendly footwear options are widely available, ensuring ethical and compassionate choices.

4. **Temperature Awareness:** Be mindful of temperature when washing your feet, ensuring that water is not too hot to avoid burns. Neuropathy can reduce temperature sensitivity, making it crucial to check water temperatures.

2. *Eye Care and Regular Screenings*

Regular eye screenings are vital for individuals with diabetes to detect and manage potential eye complications. Vegan-friendly strategies encompass specific nutrients and practices that contribute to eye health.

1. **Antioxidant-Rich Diet:** Adopt an antioxidant-rich diet, including fruits, vegetables, and whole grains. Antioxidants protect the eyes from oxidative stress and support overall eye health.

2. **Regular Eye Examinations:** Schedule regular eye examinations with an optometrist or ophthalmologist. Vegan-friendly eye care professionals can provide comprehensive eye health assessments.

3. **Hydration:** Stay adequately hydrated to support eye moisture and prevent dry eyes. Proper hydration contributes to overall eye comfort and health.

4. **Blue Light Protection:** Limit exposure to excessive blue light, especially from digital screens. Consider using blue light-blocking glasses or adjusting screen settings to reduce eye strain.

Navigating vegan challenges and managing diabetes complications requires a holistic and personalized approach. By addressing potential nutritional deficiencies, proactively managing diabetes-related complications, and adopting vegan-friendly strategies for foot and eye care, individuals can enhance their overall well-being and thrive on a plant-based lifestyle. As we conclude this chapter, the following sections will delve into practical tips for day-to-day living, optimizing nutrition for specific situations, and maintaining resilience on the journey of living well with diabetes as a vegan.

Chapter 10:

Emotional Well-being and Mindfulness for Vegans with Diabetes

Maintaining emotional well-being is integral to living a fulfilling life with diabetes, and a vegan lifestyle can offer unique avenues for fostering mindfulness and resilience. This chapter explores strategies for cultivating a positive mindset, incorporating mindful eating and stress reduction techniques, and building a supportive vegan community for emotional well-being.

Cultivating a Positive Mindset and Coping with Diabetes

Living with diabetes presents daily challenges that can impact emotional well-being. Cultivating a positive mindset is a powerful tool for coping with diabetes, promoting mental health, and enhancing overall quality of life.

1. Understanding and Acceptance

Acceptance is a cornerstone of cultivating a positive mindset when living with diabetes. Acknowledge the diagnosis, understand its implications, and embrace the journey towards effective management.

1. **Acknowledging Emotions:** It's normal to experience a range of emotions after a diabetes diagnosis. Allow yourself to feel and process these emotions, whether it's frustration, fear, or sadness. Recognizing and acknowledging these feelings is a crucial step in the journey.

2. **Educational Empowerment:** Knowledge is empowering. Learn about diabetes, its management, and the role of

a vegan lifestyle. Understanding how food choices, exercise, and other lifestyle factors impact blood sugar levels contributes to a sense of control and empowerment.

3. **Embracing Change:** Diabetes often requires lifestyle adjustments. Embrace these changes as part of a journey towards better health. Instead of viewing them as restrictions, consider them as opportunities to enhance well-being.

2. *Mindfulness and Positive Affirmations*

Mindfulness practices can significantly contribute to a positive mindset. Incorporate techniques such as meditation, deep breathing, and positive affirmations into daily life.

1. **Mindful Breathing:** Take moments throughout the day to engage in mindful breathing exercises. Focus on your breath, inhaling and exhaling slowly. This simple practice can help reduce stress and bring a sense of calm.

2. **Meditation for Stress Reduction:** Explore meditation practices designed to reduce stress and promote relaxation. Guided meditations or mindfulness apps can be valuable resources for incorporating meditation into daily routines.

3. **Positive Affirmations:** Affirmations are positive statements that reinforce a constructive mindset. Create personalized affirmations related to diabetes management and overall well-being. Repeat these affirmations regularly to foster a positive internal dialogue.

3. *Setting Realistic Goals and Celebrating Achievements*

Establishing realistic goals and celebrating achievements, no matter how small, contributes to a positive mindset. Break larger objectives into manageable steps and acknowledge progress along the way.

1. **SMART Goals:** Use the SMART criteria (Specific, Measurable, Achievable, Relevant, Time-bound) when setting goals related to diabetes management and lifestyle changes. This framework enhances clarity and feasibility.

2. **Tracking Progress:** Keep a journal or use apps to track blood sugar levels, dietary choices, and physical activity. Monitoring progress provides valuable insights and allows for adjustments when necessary.

3. **Celebrating Successes:** Celebrate achievements, whether it's reaching a specific blood sugar target, consistently following a balanced vegan diet, or incorporating regular exercise. Positive reinforcement strengthens motivation and resilience.

By cultivating a positive mindset, individuals with diabetes can navigate challenges with resilience, focus on progress, and enhance their emotional well-being.

Mindful Eating and Stress Reduction Techniques for Vegans

Mindful eating and stress reduction techniques are essential components of emotional well-being for individuals with diabetes. Incorporating these practices into a vegan lifestyle can contribute to a harmonious relationship with food, improved blood sugar control, and reduced stress.

1. *Mindful Eating Practices*

Mindful eating involves paying full attention to the sensory experience of eating, fostering a deeper connection with food, and promoting healthier eating habits.

1. **Savoring Each Bite:** Take the time to savor each bite, appreciating the flavors, textures, and aromas of the food. Eating slowly and mindfully allows for better digestion and enhances the overall dining experience.

2. **Engaging the Senses:** Engage all your senses during meals. Notice the colors, smells, and textures of your food. This heightened awareness fosters a greater appreciation for the nourishment provided by each meal.

3. **Listening to Hunger Cues:** Pay attention to hunger and fullness cues. Eat when you're hungry and stop when you're satisfied. Mindful eating helps prevent overeating and promotes a balanced approach to nutrition.

2. *Stress Reduction Techniques*

Stress can impact blood sugar levels, making stress reduction techniques crucial for individuals with diabetes. Vegan-friendly stress reduction practices contribute to emotional well-being and overall health.

1. **Breathing Exercises:** Practice deep breathing exercises to activate the body's relaxation response. Slow, intentional breaths can alleviate stress and promote a sense of calm.

2. **Yoga and Stretching:** Incorporate gentle yoga or stretching into your routine. These practices not only reduce physical tension but also contribute to mental relaxation.

3. **Nature Connection:** Spend time in nature to recharge and reduce stress. Whether it's a walk in a park, gardening, or simply enjoying outdoor scenery, nature has a calming effect on the mind.

3. *Mind-Body Connection and Intuitive Eating*

The mind-body connection plays a significant role in emotional well-being and can influence eating behaviors. Intuitive eating, rooted in the mind-body connection, emphasizes listening to the body's cues for nourishment.

1. **Listening to Hunger and Fullness:** Tune in to your body's signals for hunger and fullness. Avoid restrictive eating patterns and trust your body's innate ability to guide your nutritional needs.

2. **Emotional Eating Awareness:** Be mindful of emotional eating triggers. Identifying emotional cues for eating allows for more conscious choices, promoting a healthier relationship with food.

3. **Gratitude Practice:** Cultivate a gratitude practice related to food. Express gratitude for the nourishment provided by each meal, fostering a positive and appreciative mindset towards food choices.

By integrating mindful eating practices and stress reduction techniques into a vegan lifestyle, individuals with diabetes can enhance their overall emotional well-being and create a more balanced approach to nutrition.

The journey of living well with diabetes is often more manageable and fulfilling when shared with a supportive community. Building a vegan community that understands the unique challenges of managing diabetes fosters emotional support, camaraderie, and shared wisdom.

1. *Online Vegan Communities and Forums*

Online platforms provide an invaluable space for connecting with like-minded individuals who share both a vegan lifestyle and the experience of living with diabetes.

1. **Social Media Groups:** Join vegan and diabetes-related groups on social media platforms. These groups often offer a platform for asking questions, sharing experiences, and gaining insights from others on a similar journey.

2. **Vegan Diabetes Blogs:** Explore blogs and websites dedicated to the intersection of veganism and diabetes. Many individuals share their personal stories, tips, and recipes, creating a sense of community and encouragement.

3. **Virtual Events and Webinars:** Attend virtual events and webinars focused on veganism and diabetes. These gatherings provide opportunities to learn, connect with experts, and engage with a supportive community.

2. *Local Vegan Meetups and Events*

Connecting with local vegan communities adds a personal dimension to the support network, fostering real-world relationships and shared experiences.

1. **Vegan Meetup Groups:** Join local vegan meetup groups or create one in your community. These groups can organize events, potlucks, and activities that provide opportunities for socializing and support.

2. **Plant-Based Cooking Classes:** Attend or organize plant-based cooking classes or workshops in your area. Sharing culinary experiences with others fosters a sense of community and provides practical insights into vegan meal preparation.

3. **Community Gardens:** Engage in community gardening initiatives. Growing and sharing plant-based foods with others not only supports a sustainable lifestyle but also creates bonds within the vegan community.

3. *Vegan Support Networks for Diabetes*

Specialized support networks that focus on both veganism and diabetes offer a targeted and understanding community.

1. **Diabetes Support Groups:** Explore or establish diabetes support groups that specifically cater to individuals following a vegan lifestyle. These groups can discuss vegan-friendly strategies for diabetes management and offer emotional support.

2. **Vegan Retreats and Events:** Attend vegan retreats or events that incorporate discussions on managing diabetes. These gatherings bring together individuals with shared values and experiences in a supportive environment.

3. **Collaborative Initiatives:** Collaborate with local healthcare professionals, nutritionists, and vegan advocates to organize initiatives focused on diabetes awareness within the vegan community.

In summary, building a supportive vegan community enhances emotional well-being by creating a network of understanding individuals who share similar values and experiences. The exchange of knowledge, encouragement, and camaraderie within this community contributes to a positive and resilient mindset in the face of the challenges associated with diabetes.

As we conclude this chapter, it's evident that emotional well-being is an integral aspect of living well with diabetes as a vegan. By cultivating a positive mindset, incorporating mindful eating and stress reduction techniques, and building a supportive vegan community, individuals can navigate the emotional aspects of diabetes with resilience, compassion, and a sense of shared purpose. The subsequent chapters will delve into practical tips for daily living, optimizing nutrition for specific situations, and maintaining long-term well-being on the journey of living better with diabetes as a vegan.

Chapter 11:

Veganism and Diabetes Prevention

Veganism, with its focus on plant-based nutrition, offers a powerful approach to preventing type 2 diabetes and promoting overall health. This chapter explores the role of a vegan lifestyle in preventing diabetes, the connection between weight management and diabetes risk reduction for vegans, and strategies for promoting long-term health through a vegan approach.

Preventing Type 2 Diabetes through a Vegan Lifestyle

Type 2 diabetes is a preventable and manageable condition, and adopting a vegan lifestyle can be a proactive step towards reducing the risk of developing this prevalent metabolic disorder.

1. *Plant-Based Nutrition for Diabetes Prevention*

A vegan diet centered around whole, plant-based foods provides numerous health benefits, making it an effective tool in preventing type 2 diabetes.

1. **Fiber-Rich Foods:** Plant-based diets naturally include high-fiber foods such as fruits, vegetables, whole grains, legumes, and nuts. Fiber plays a crucial role in stabilizing blood sugar levels and improving insulin sensitivity, key factors in diabetes prevention.

2. **Low-Glycemic Index Foods:** Many plant-based foods have a low glycemic index, meaning they cause a slower and more gradual increase in blood sugar levels. This can help prevent spikes and crashes, promoting stable glucose levels.

3. **Reduced Saturated Fat:** A vegan diet typically contains lower levels of saturated fat, found predominantly in animal products. Lowering saturated fat intake contributes to improved insulin sensitivity and a reduced risk of type 2 diabetes.

2. Antioxidants and Phytochemicals

Plant-based foods are rich in antioxidants and phytochemicals, compounds that play a vital role in preventing cellular damage and inflammation, both of which are associated with the development of diabetes.

1. **Colorful Fruits and Vegetables:** Vibrantly colored fruits and vegetables are rich in antioxidants like vitamins A, C, and E, as well as phytochemicals. These compounds protect cells from oxidative stress and inflammation.

2. **Herbs and Spices:** Many herbs and spices, such as turmeric, cinnamon, and ginger, have anti-inflammatory and antioxidant properties. Incorporating these into a vegan diet adds flavor while supporting overall health.

3. **Whole Plant Foods:** Consuming a variety of whole plant foods ensures a diverse intake of antioxidants and phytochemicals. This diversity contributes to overall health and helps prevent chronic conditions like type 2 diabetes.

3. Maintaining a Healthy Weight

Weight management is a crucial aspect of diabetes prevention, and a vegan lifestyle provides a framework for achieving and maintaining a healthy weight.

1. **Plant-Based Weight Loss:** Numerous studies have shown that adopting a vegan diet can be effective for weight loss. The emphasis on whole, nutrient-dense foods often leads to reduced calorie intake while still providing essential nutrients.

2. **Increased Fiber and Satiety:** The high fiber content in plant-based diets promotes feelings of fullness and satiety. This can lead to better portion control and reduced overeating, supporting weight management efforts.

3. **Plant-Based Protein Sources:** Plant-based protein sources, such as legumes, tofu, tempeh, and seitan, contribute to muscle maintenance and growth while often containing fewer calories and less saturated fat compared to animal-based protein sources.

4. *Blood Sugar Control and Insulin Sensitivity*

A vegan lifestyle supports optimal blood sugar control and insulin sensitivity, key factors in preventing type 2 diabetes.

1. **Carbohydrate Quality:** Whole plant foods provide complex carbohydrates that are slowly digested, leading to a gradual release of glucose into the bloodstream. This supports stable blood sugar levels and reduces the risk of insulin resistance.

2. **Healthy Fats:** Plant-based fats, such as those found in avocados, nuts, seeds, and olive oil, contribute to overall health and can improve insulin sensitivity. Choosing healthy fats in a vegan diet supports diabetes prevention.

3. **Avoiding Animal-Based Insulin Resistance Factors:** Animal-based products, particularly those high in saturated fat, have been linked to insulin resistance. By avoiding these factors, a vegan diet helps maintain insulin sensitivity.

In conclusion, preventing type 2 diabetes through a vegan lifestyle involves adopting a plant-based diet rich in fiber, antioxidants, and phytochemicals. This dietary approach, coupled with the benefits of weight management, blood sugar control, and improved insulin sensitivity, creates a holistic strategy for reducing the risk of developing diabetes.

Weight Management and Diabetes Risk Reduction for Vegans

Weight management plays a pivotal role in reducing the risk of developing type 2 diabetes, and a vegan lifestyle provides a favorable environment for achieving and maintaining a healthy weight.

1. *Plant-Based Nutrition and Weight Control*

A vegan diet offers a wealth of nutrient-dense, low-calorie foods that support weight control and contribute to overall well-being.

1. **High-Fiber Foods:** Plant-based diets are naturally rich in fiber, promoting feelings of fullness and reducing overall calorie intake. Fiber also supports digestive health and contributes to long-term weight management.

2. **Low-Calorie Density:** Many plant-based foods have low-calorie density, meaning they provide fewer calories per gram. This allows individuals to consume larger volumes

of food while managing calorie intake, making it easier to achieve and maintain a healthy weight.

3. **Whole Foods Focus:** Emphasizing whole, minimally processed foods in a vegan diet ensures a nutrient-dense approach to eating. Whole foods provide essential vitamins, minerals, and antioxidants without excessive calories, supporting weight management.

2. Plant-Based Protein and Satiety

Protein plays a crucial role in satiety and muscle maintenance, and a vegan diet offers a variety of plant-based protein sources.

1. **Legumes and Pulses:** Beans, lentils, and chickpeas are excellent sources of plant-based protein. They not only contribute to satiety but also provide a range of nutrients and fiber.

2. **Tofu and Tempeh:** Soy-based products like tofu and tempeh are versatile protein sources that can be incorporated into a variety of dishes. These options support muscle health and aid in weight management.

3. **Nuts and Seeds:** Including nuts and seeds in the diet provides healthy fats, protein, and fiber. They are satisfying snacks that contribute to satiety and can be part of a balanced approach to weight management.

3. Balanced Macronutrients for Weight Stability

Achieving and maintaining a healthy weight involves a balanced intake of macronutrients, and a vegan lifestyle offers a natural balance.

1. **Carbohydrates for Energy:** Whole grains, fruits, and vegetables provide complex carbohydrates that serve as

the body's primary energy source. Choosing whole, unprocessed carbs supports sustained energy levels and weight stability.

2. **Healthy Fats for Satiety:** Including sources of healthy fats, such as avocados, olives, and nuts, contributes to satiety. These fats provide essential nutrients and add flavor to meals without compromising weight management.

3. **Protein for Muscle Maintenance:** A sufficient intake of plant-based protein supports muscle maintenance and growth. This is crucial for weight management, as muscle mass plays a role in overall metabolic health.

4. *Portion Control and Mindful Eating*

Adopting mindful eating practices and paying attention to portion sizes are fundamental aspects of weight management within a vegan lifestyle.

1. **Mindful Eating Techniques:** Engage in mindful eating by paying attention to hunger and fullness cues. Avoid distractions during meals, savor each bite, and listen to your body's signals to prevent overeating.

2. **Balanced Meals and Snacks:** Plan balanced meals and snacks that include a mix of macronutrients. This approach supports satiety, preventing excessive calorie intake and contributing to weight stability.

3. **Hydration and Appetite Regulation:** Stay adequately hydrated, as thirst can sometimes be mistaken for hunger. Drinking water before meals can help regulate appetite and prevent overeating.

By embracing a vegan lifestyle and focusing on nutrient-dense, plant-based foods, individuals can naturally support weight management and reduce the risk of developing type 2 diabetes.

Promoting Long-Term Health with a Vegan Approach

A vegan lifestyle not only aids in preventing type 2 diabetes but also contributes to long-term health and well-being. This section explores the holistic benefits of a vegan approach beyond diabetes prevention.

1. *Heart Health and Cholesterol Management*

A vegan diet has been associated with numerous cardiovascular benefits, including lower cholesterol levels, reduced blood pressure, and a decreased risk of heart disease.

1. **Low Saturated Fat Intake:** Vegan diets are typically low in saturated fat, which is known to raise cholesterol levels. By avoiding animal products, individuals reduce their intake of saturated fats, promoting heart health.

2. **Rich in Heart-Healthy Nutrients:** Plant-based diets provide an abundance of heart-healthy nutrients, such as fiber, antioxidants, and omega-3 fatty acids. These nutrients contribute to cardiovascular well-being and overall longevity.

3. **Reduced Risk of Hypertension:** The emphasis on whole, plant-based foods in a vegan diet supports healthy blood pressure levels, reducing the risk of hypertension and its associated complications.

2. *Cancer Prevention and Plant-Based Diets*

Certain aspects of a vegan lifestyle have been linked to a reduced risk of various types of cancer.

1. **Antioxidant-Rich Foods:** The high intake of antioxidants from fruits, vegetables, and other plant-based sources helps protect cells from oxidative stress, potentially reducing the risk of certain cancers.

2. **Phytochemicals and Cancer Protection:** Phytochemicals found in plant-based foods have been studied for their potential anti-cancer properties. These compounds may play a role in preventing the development and progression of certain cancers.

3. **Avoidance of Processed and Red Meats:** Vegan diets exclude processed and red meats, which have been associated with an increased risk of colorectal and other cancers. Choosing plant-based alternatives reduces exposure to these risk factors.

3. Bone Health and Vegan Nutrition

Contrary to some misconceptions, a well-planned vegan diet can support optimal bone health and reduce the risk of osteoporosis.

1. **Calcium-Rich Plant Foods:** Many plant-based foods, including fortified plant milk, tofu, leafy greens, and almonds, are rich in calcium. Incorporating these into the diet supports bone health without relying on dairy products.

2. **Vitamin D Synthesis:** Exposure to sunlight stimulates the synthesis of vitamin D in the skin. A vegan lifestyle encourages outdoor activities, contributing to natural vitamin D production and supporting bone health.

3. **Balanced Nutrient Intake:** A well-rounded vegan diet includes a variety of nutrients, such as vitamin K,

magnesium, and potassium, which contribute to overall bone health. Ensuring a balanced nutrient intake is essential for long-term well-being.

4. *Anti-Inflammatory Effects of Vegan Nutrition*

Chronic inflammation is linked to various chronic diseases, and a vegan lifestyle can have anti-inflammatory effects, promoting long-term health.

1. **Omega-3 Fatty Acids:** Plant-based sources of omega-3 fatty acids, such as flaxseeds, chia seeds, and walnuts, contribute to an anti-inflammatory diet. Balancing the ratio of omega-3 to omega-6 fatty acids is essential for managing inflammation.

2. **Colorful Fruits and Vegetables:** The vibrant colors of fruits and vegetables are indicative of their rich antioxidant content, which helps combat inflammation. Including a variety of colorful plant foods in the diet supports overall health.

3. **Avoidance of Pro-Inflammatory Foods:** A vegan lifestyle typically excludes pro-inflammatory foods like processed meats and certain dairy products. This dietary choice reduces exposure to substances that can contribute to inflammation.

Summarily then, a vegan approach not only prevents type 2 diabetes but also promotes long-term health and well-being. By emphasizing heart health, reducing the risk of cancer, supporting bone health, and adopting an anti-inflammatory diet, individuals can thrive on a plant-based journey toward a healthier and more fulfilling life. As we conclude this chapter, the subsequent sections will provide practical insights for daily living, optimizing nutrition for specific situations, and maintaining resilience on the journey of living better with diabetes as a vegan.

Chapter 12:

Thriving as a Vegan with Diabetes

Thriving as a vegan with diabetes involves celebrating successes, overcoming challenges, advocating for vegan-friendly diabetes care, and empowering both yourself and others in the vegan community. This chapter explores the importance of acknowledging achievements, navigating obstacles, influencing positive change in diabetes care, and fostering a supportive community that empowers and inspires.

Celebrating Successes and Overcoming Challenges

Celebrating successes and overcoming challenges is a dynamic aspect of thriving as a vegan with diabetes. Acknowledging achievements, no matter how small, contributes to a positive mindset and resilience on this unique journey.

1. *Setting Personal Milestones and Acknowledging Progress*

Setting personal milestones is an empowering practice that allows individuals to establish tangible goals and celebrate their achievements.

1. **Blood Sugar Management:** Establish milestones related to blood sugar levels, such as achieving and maintaining target ranges. Celebrate successes in stabilizing glucose levels through lifestyle changes and dietary choices.

2. **Physical Activity Goals:** Set goals for physical activity and celebrate accomplishments in maintaining an active lifestyle. Whether it's walking, jogging, or engaging in specific exercises, tracking progress enhances motivation.

3. **Nutritional Achievements:** Acknowledge milestones in adopting a balanced and nutritious vegan diet. Celebrate diversifying food choices, incorporating new recipes, and mastering the art of crafting well-balanced meals.

2. Mindset Shifts and Positive Habits

Thriving with diabetes involves cultivating a positive mindset and establishing healthy habits that contribute to overall well-being.

1. **Mindfulness Practices:** Celebrate the incorporation of mindfulness practices into daily life. Whether it's mindful eating, meditation, or gratitude exercises, recognize the positive impact on mental and emotional health.

2. **Consistent Self-Care:** Acknowledge the establishment of consistent self-care routines. Celebrate the commitment to regular blood sugar monitoring, medication management, and other aspects of diabetes care.

3. **Building Resilience:** Recognize the development of resilience in the face of challenges. Celebrate the ability to bounce back from setbacks, learn from experiences, and adapt to the evolving nature of diabetes management.

3. Overcoming Vegan-Specific Challenges

Navigating challenges unique to a vegan lifestyle with diabetes requires resilience and creative problem-solving.

1. **Social Situations:** Celebrate successful navigation of social gatherings and events while adhering to a vegan diet and managing diabetes. Share experiences and strategies with the vegan community to inspire others facing similar challenges.

2. **Dining Out:** Acknowledge accomplishments in making informed choices when dining out at restaurants. Celebrate the ability to communicate dietary needs effectively and enjoy vegan-friendly options while maintaining blood sugar control.

3. **Traveling as a Vegan with Diabetes:** Recognize successful travel experiences as a vegan with diabetes. Celebrate the ability to plan and prepare for travel, ensuring access to suitable food options and managing diabetes care away from home.

Celebrating successes, whether related to blood sugar management, mindset shifts, or overcoming vegan-specific challenges, reinforces a positive approach to living well with diabetes as a vegan.

Advocating for Vegan-Friendly Diabetes Care

Advocacy is a powerful tool for influencing positive change in diabetes care, ensuring that healthcare systems and providers are knowledgeable and supportive of vegan lifestyles.

1. Promoting Vegan-Friendly Healthcare Practices

Advocating for vegan-friendly healthcare practices involves raising awareness among healthcare professionals and promoting inclusive care for individuals with diabetes.

1. **Educating Healthcare Providers:** Advocate for the education of healthcare providers about the benefits

and challenges of a vegan lifestyle in diabetes management. Encourage workshops, seminars, or informational materials to enhance their understanding.

2. **Inclusive Diabetes Education:** Promote the development of inclusive diabetes education materials that specifically address the needs of individuals following a vegan diet. This ensures that dietary recommendations align with ethical choices and preferences.

3. **Collaborating with Diabetes Organizations:** Advocate for collaboration between diabetes organizations and vegan advocacy groups. This collaboration can lead to the creation of resources, support networks, and events that cater to the intersection of veganism and diabetes.

2. *Influencing Policy Changes for Vegan-Friendly Care*

Advocacy efforts can extend to influencing policy changes that support vegan-friendly diabetes care within healthcare institutions.

1. **Policy Recommendations:** Develop and propose policy recommendations that promote vegan-friendly care. This may include guidelines for accommodating vegan dietary preferences, updating meal plans, and integrating plant-based nutrition into diabetes management protocols.

2. **Collaborating with Nutrition Departments:** Advocate for collaboration between healthcare institutions and nutrition departments to ensure the availability of

vegan-friendly options in hospitals, clinics, and other healthcare settings.

3. **Vegan-Friendly Meal Planning in Healthcare Settings:** Work towards the inclusion of vegan-friendly meal planning options in healthcare settings. This can involve collaborating with nutritionists and chefs to create diverse and nutritionally balanced plant-based meal options.

3. *Community Engagement and Education*

Community engagement plays a crucial role in advocating for vegan-friendly diabetes care. Empowering individuals with knowledge and resources fosters a sense of agency in managing their health.

1. **Community Workshops and Seminars:** Organize workshops and seminars within the vegan community to educate individuals about diabetes management. Provide information on blood sugar control, nutrition, and the intersection of veganism and diabetes.

2. **Online Resources and Support Groups:** Establish online resources and support groups that focus on vegan-friendly diabetes care. These platforms can serve as spaces for sharing experiences, seeking advice, and fostering a sense of community among individuals navigating similar journeys.

3. **Collaboration with Vegan Influencers:** Collaborate with vegan influencers and advocates to amplify the message of vegan-friendly diabetes care. Influencers can use their platforms to share information, personal stories,

and resources that empower their followers with diabetes.

By actively advocating for vegan-friendly diabetes care, individuals contribute to a more inclusive and supportive healthcare environment that aligns with their ethical choices and dietary preferences.

Empowering oneself and inspiring others within the vegan community involves sharing knowledge, building resilience, and fostering a supportive network.

1. *Continuous Learning and Personal Growth*

Empowering oneself in the vegan community with diabetes requires a commitment to continuous learning and personal growth.

1. **Staying Informed:** Engage in ongoing research and stay informed about advancements in diabetes management, nutrition, and vegan-friendly resources. This knowledge empowers individuals to make informed decisions about their health.

2. **Attending Workshops and Webinars:** Participate in workshops, webinars, and events focused on diabetes management within the vegan lifestyle. These educational opportunities provide valuable insights and connect individuals with like-minded peers.

3. **Networking with Healthcare Professionals:** Build connections with healthcare professionals who understand and support vegan lifestyles. Collaborate

with dietitians, endocrinologists, and other specialists who can provide personalized guidance for diabetes care.

2. *Sharing Personal Experiences and Success Stories*

Sharing personal experiences and success stories within the vegan community creates a supportive and inspiring environment.

1. **Blogging and Social Media:** Consider sharing your journey through blogs, social media, or other online platforms. Discuss your experiences, challenges, and triumphs as a vegan managing diabetes to inspire and connect with others.

2. **Participating in Vegan Events:** Attend vegan events, conferences, and gatherings to share your story with a broader audience. Networking at these events can lead to meaningful connections and the exchange of valuable insights.

3. **Collaborating with Vegan Organizations:** Collaborate with vegan organizations to share your experiences in their publications or events. Your story can serve as inspiration for others navigating a vegan lifestyle with diabetes.

3. *Fostering Supportive Networks within the Vegan Community*

Building supportive networks within the vegan community involves creating spaces for mutual encouragement, understanding, and inspiration.

1. **Local Meetups and Events:** Organize or participate in local meetups and events for vegans with diabetes. These gatherings provide opportunities for face-to-face connections, shared experiences, and valuable support.

2. **Online Support Groups:** Contribute to online support groups dedicated to veganism and diabetes. Actively participate in discussions, offer advice, and share resources to create a sense of community among members.

3. **Collaborative Initiatives:** Explore collaborative initiatives within the vegan community to promote health and well-being. This could involve partnering with local businesses, healthcare professionals, and vegan advocates to organize events or initiatives focused on diabetes management.

Thriving as a vegan with diabetes is a multi-faceted journey that involves celebrating successes, advocating for vegan-friendly diabetes care, and empowering oneself and others within the vegan community. By setting personal milestones, influencing positive change in healthcare practices, and fostering a supportive network, individuals can navigate the challenges and triumphs of living well with diabetes as a vegan. The subsequent chapters will delve into practical tips for daily living, optimizing nutrition for specific situations, and maintaining resilience on the journey of living better with diabetes as a vegan.

Conclusion:

Living a Vibrant and Healthy Life with Diabetes as a Vegan

Embarking on the journey of living a vibrant and healthy life with diabetes as a vegan is a testament to the resilience, commitment, and empowerment of individuals who have chosen this unique path. This holistic approach to health encompasses not only the intricacies of managing diabetes but also the ethical and compassionate choice of adopting a vegan lifestyle. As we conclude this guide, let's reflect on the key principles and insights that can pave the way for a fulfilling and sustainable life.

Celebrating the Symbiosis of Veganism and Diabetes Management

Living vibrantly with diabetes as a vegan is not just about managing blood sugar levels; it's a celebration of the symbiosis between compassionate living and optimal health. The chapters explored the profound impact of a plant-based diet on diabetes prevention, blood sugar control, and overall well-being. By embracing the power of plant-based nutrition, individuals have unlocked a wealth of benefits, from improved insulin sensitivity to enhanced heart health, reinforcing the idea that vibrant living is achievable through mindful dietary choices.

Crafting a Nutrient-Dense Vegan Lifestyle

Crafting a nutrient-dense vegan lifestyle emerged as a cornerstone of this journey. From understanding the types of diabetes and its prevalence within the vegan community to addressing nutritional concerns and exploring vegan-friendly alternatives, each chapter unfolded layers of knowledge. The emphasis on key nutrients, balanced meal planning, and smart shopping underscored the importance of informed choices in nourishing the body and mind. This knowledge empowers individuals to navigate the complexities of diabetes management while thriving on a plant-based diet.

Practical Insights for Daily Living

The guide delved into practical insights for daily living, acknowledging the challenges unique to the intersection of veganism and diabetes. From navigating social situations and dining out to mastering meal planning and cooking techniques, the content provided real-world strategies. These insights extend beyond the theoretical, offering tangible solutions for individuals to integrate into their daily lives. By understanding the nuances of living as a vegan with diabetes, individuals can confidently navigate diverse scenarios, fostering a sense of control and well-being.

Building a Supportive Vegan Community

A recurring theme throughout the guide emphasized the importance of building a supportive vegan community. The chapters explored the role of community in emotional well-being, navigating challenges, and inspiring positive change. The collaborative efforts of individuals, whether through local meetups, online support groups, or advocacy initiatives, contribute to a sense of belonging and shared purpose. In the face of potential nutritional concerns and diabetes complications, a supportive community becomes a pillar of strength, offering encouragement, understanding, and valuable insights.

Empowerment, Advocacy, and Inspiration

Thriving as a vegan with diabetes involves empowerment, advocacy, and inspiration. By setting personal milestones, advocating for vegan-friendly healthcare practices, and sharing experiences within the vegan community, individuals become architects of their health journey. The guide encouraged continuous learning, personal growth, and the empowerment of oneself and others. As advocates for change, individuals play a crucial role in influencing healthcare practices, and policy changes, and promoting inclusivity for those managing diabetes within the vegan lifestyle.

Looking Forward: A Roadmap for Sustainable Well-Being

As we conclude this exploration into living better with diabetes as a vegan, it's essential to view the insights provided as a roadmap for sustainable well-being. This guide serves as a companion, offering guidance on nutrition, lifestyle choices, and emotional resilience. It recognizes that the journey is dynamic, with its share of victories and challenges. The key lies in the ability to adapt, learn, and thrive, supported by the foundation of a plant-based lifestyle.

In the tapestry of living vibrantly with diabetes as a vegan, each individual contributes a unique thread, weaving a narrative of resilience, health, and compassion. By embracing the principles outlined in this guide, individuals can stride confidently towards a future where diabetes is managed effectively, well-being is prioritized, and the vibrancy of life is celebrated daily. May this journey be not just a response to a diagnosis but a proactive choice for a fulfilling, vibrant, and healthy existence, proving that living well with diabetes as a vegan is not only possible but profoundly enriching.

Appendix:

Vegan Recipes and Meal Ideas for Diabetes Management

Incorporating delicious and nutritious plant-based meals into your daily routine is a key aspect of managing diabetes as a vegan. The following recipes and meal ideas are designed to provide inspiration, flavor, and balanced nutrition while supporting blood sugar control. Remember to tailor portion sizes and ingredients to meet your individual dietary needs.

1. Quinoa and Vegetable Stir-Fry:

Ingredients:

- 1 cup quinoa, cooked

- 2 cups mixed vegetables (broccoli, bell peppers, carrots, snap peas)

- 1 tablespoon low-sodium soy sauce

- 1 tablespoon sesame oil

- 1 clove garlic, minced

- 1 teaspoon fresh ginger, grated

- 2 green onions, chopped

- Sesame seeds for garnish

Instructions:

1. In a wok or large skillet, heat sesame oil over medium-high heat.

2. Add garlic and ginger, and sauté for 1-2 minutes until fragrant.

3. Add mixed vegetables and stir-fry until they are crisp-tender.

4. Stir in cooked quinoa and soy sauce, tossing to combine.

5. Cook for an additional 2-3 minutes until everything is heated through.

6. Garnish with chopped green onions and sesame seeds.

2. Lentil and Vegetable Soup:

Ingredients:

- 1 cup dry green or brown lentils, rinsed

- 1 onion, diced

- 2 carrots, diced

- 2 celery stalks, diced

- 3 cloves garlic, minced

- 1 can (14 oz) diced tomatoes

- 6 cups vegetable broth

- 1 teaspoon cumin

- 1 teaspoon smoked paprika

- Salt and pepper to taste

- Fresh parsley for garnish

Instructions:

1. In a large pot, sauté onions, carrots, celery, and garlic until softened.

2. Add lentils, diced tomatoes, vegetable broth, cumin, smoked paprika, salt, and pepper.

3. Bring the soup to a boil, then reduce heat and let it simmer for 25-30 minutes until lentils are tender.

4. Adjust seasoning as needed.

5. Garnish with fresh parsley before serving.

3. Chickpea and Spinach Curry:

Ingredients:

- 1 can (15 oz) chickpeas, drained and rinsed

- 1 onion, finely chopped

- 2 tomatoes, diced

- 3 cups fresh spinach

- 1 can (14 oz) coconut milk

- 2 tablespoons curry powder

- 1 teaspoon turmeric

- 1 teaspoon cumin

- Salt and pepper to taste

- Fresh cilantro for garnish

Instructions:

1. In a large skillet, sauté chopped onion until translucent.

2. Add curry powder, turmeric, and cumin, stirring for 1-2 minutes.

3. Add diced tomatoes and cook until softened.

4. Stir in chickpeas and coconut milk, and simmer for 10-15 minutes.

5. Add fresh spinach and cook until wilted.

6. Season with salt and pepper, garnish with fresh cilantro.

4. Baked Stuffed Bell Peppers:

Ingredients:

- 4 large bell peppers, halved and seeds removed

- 1 cup quinoa, cooked

- 1 can (15 oz) black beans, drained and rinsed

- 1 cup corn kernels (fresh or frozen)

- 1 cup salsa

- 1 teaspoon cumin

- 1 teaspoon chili powder

- 1 cup vegan cheese, shredded (optional)

- Fresh cilantro for garnish

Instructions:

1. Preheat the oven to 375°F (190°C).

2. In a bowl, mix cooked quinoa, black beans, corn, salsa, cumin, and chili powder.

3. Stuff each bell pepper half with the quinoa mixture.

4. Place the stuffed peppers in a baking dish and cover with foil.

5. Bake for 25-30 minutes until peppers are tender.

6. If desired, sprinkle vegan cheese on top and bake for an additional 5 minutes.

7. Garnish with fresh cilantro before serving.

5. Berry and Chia Seed Pudding:

Ingredients:

- 1/4 cup chia seeds

- 1 cup almond milk

- 1 teaspoon vanilla extract

- 1 tablespoon maple syrup

- Mixed berries (strawberries, blueberries, raspberries)

Instructions:

1. In a jar, mix chia seeds, almond milk, vanilla extract, and maple syrup.

2. Stir well and refrigerate for at least 4 hours or overnight.

3. Before serving, stir the chia pudding to ensure a smooth consistency.

4. Layer the chia pudding with mixed berries in a serving glass.

5. Garnish with additional berries on top.

These recipes offer a variety of flavors, textures, and nutrients to keep your meals exciting while supporting your vegan lifestyle and diabetes management. Experiment with these ideas, and don't hesitate to modify them according to your preferences and nutritional needs. Enjoy the journey of creating vibrant and delicious meals that contribute to your overall well-being.

Glossary:

Key Terms Related to Diabetes and Veganism

Understanding the terminology associated with diabetes and veganism is essential for navigating the complexities of managing health within the context of a plant-based lifestyle. This glossary provides definitions for key terms to enhance your comprehension of the intersection between diabetes and vegan living.

A1C (Glycated Hemoglobin): A blood test that measures the average blood glucose levels over the past two to three months. It is a crucial indicator for assessing long-term blood sugar control in individuals with diabetes.

Beta Cells: Cells in the pancreas responsible for producing insulin, a hormone essential for regulating blood sugar levels.

Blood Glucose: The concentration of glucose (sugar) present in the bloodstream. Monitoring blood glucose levels is vital for individuals with diabetes to manage their condition.

Carbohydrate Counting: A method of meal planning for diabetes management that involves tracking the number of carbohydrates consumed, as they directly impact blood sugar levels.

Insulin Resistance: A condition where cells do not respond effectively to insulin, leading to elevated blood glucose levels. It is a characteristic feature of type 2 diabetes.

Ketosis: A metabolic state where the body utilizes fat for energy instead of carbohydrates. It can occur in individuals with diabetes, particularly those with type 1 diabetes if insulin levels are insufficient.

Low-Glycemic Index (GI): A measure of how quickly a food raises blood sugar levels. Foods with a low glycemic index are digested more slowly, resulting in a gradual and steady increase in blood glucose.

Macronutrients: Essential nutrients that provide energy to the body. The three main macronutrients are carbohydrates, proteins, and fats.

Microvascular Complications: Diabetes-related complications that affect small blood vessels, including those in the eyes (retinopathy), kidneys (nephropathy), and nerves (neuropathy).

Neuropathy: Nerve damage that can result from uncontrolled diabetes. Symptoms may include pain, tingling, or numbness, often affecting the extremities.

Plant-Based Diet: A diet primarily composed of plant-derived foods, such as fruits, vegetables, grains, legumes, nuts, and seeds. It excludes or minimizes the consumption of animal products.

Type 1 Diabetes: A form of diabetes characterized by the immune system attacking and destroying insulin-producing beta cells in the pancreas. Individuals with type 1 diabetes require insulin therapy for survival.

Type 2 Diabetes: A common form of diabetes where the body becomes resistant to insulin, and the pancreas cannot produce enough insulin to maintain normal blood glucose levels. Lifestyle changes, including diet and exercise, are often crucial in managing type 2 diabetes.

Veganism: A lifestyle and dietary choice that abstains from the consumption of animal products, including meat, dairy, eggs, and honey. Vegans often embrace this choice for ethical, environmental, and health reasons.

Whole Foods: Unprocessed or minimally processed foods that retain their natural state and nutritional integrity. Whole foods, such as fruits, vegetables, whole grains, and legumes, are staples in a plant-based diet.

This glossary provides a foundation for understanding key terms relevant to both diabetes and veganism. As you navigate the intricacies of managing diabetes within a vegan lifestyle, familiarity with these terms will empower you to make informed decisions about your health and well-being.

9 798879 315318